Dance and the Body in Western Theatre

1948 to the Present

Sabine Sörgel

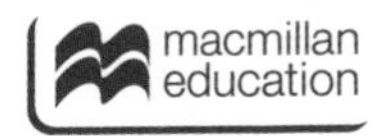

palgrave

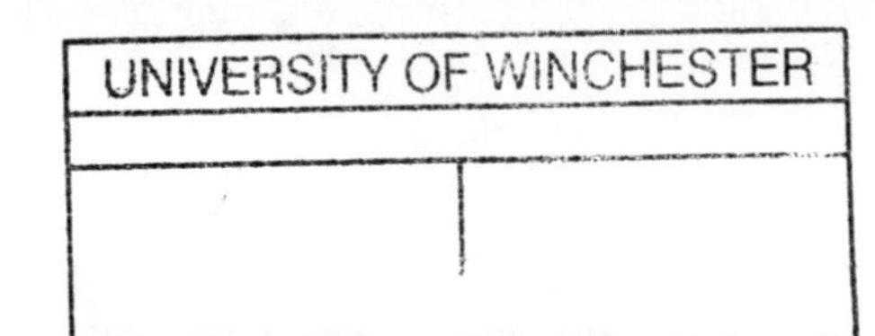

First published 2015 by
PALGRAVE

Palgrave in the UK is an imprint of Macmillan Publishers Limited, registered in England, company number 785998, of 4 Crinan Street, London, N1 9XW.

Palgrave Macmillan in the US is a division of St Martin's Press LLC, 175 Fifth Avenue, New York, NY 10010.

Palgrave is a global imprint of the above companies and is represented throughout the world.

Palgrave® and Macmillan® are registered trademarks in the United States, the United Kingdom, Europe and other countries.

ISBN 978–1–137–03488–5 hardback
ISBN 978–1–137–03487–8 paperback

This book is printed on paper suitable for recycling and made from fully managed and sustained forest sources. Logging, pulping and manufacturing processes are expected to conform to the environmental regulations of the country of origin.

A catalogue record for this book is available from the British Library.

A catalog record for this book is available from the Library of Congress.

Library of Congress Cataloging-in-Publication Data

Sörgel, Sabine.
Dance and the body in western theatre : 1948 to the present / Sabine Sörgel.
pages cm
Summary: "The mid to late twentieth century has been widely regarded as the century of the body, when philosophers, cultural critics, sociologists, and theatre historians spent inordinate amounts of time and energy locating, dissecting, and celebrating the body in performance. While the body appears in almost all cultural discourses, it is nowhere as visible or as exposed as in dance and yet dance is rarely considered in theatre histories. This book captures the resurgence of the dancing body in the aftermath of World War Two. Thought-provoking and easy to follow, the text provides students with several key phenomenological, kinaesthetic and psychological concepts relevant to both theatre and dance studies. Photographs and study questions feature at the end of each chapter, providing context for students and a starting point for further research"— Provided by publisher.
ISBN 978–1–137–03487–8 (paperback) — ISBN 978–1–137–03488–5 (paperback)
1. Theater—History—20th century. 2. Dance—History—20th century. 3. Human body—Symbolic aspects. 4. Movement, Aesthetics of. I. Title.
PN2189.S66 2015
792.0904—dc23 2015023909

Printed in China

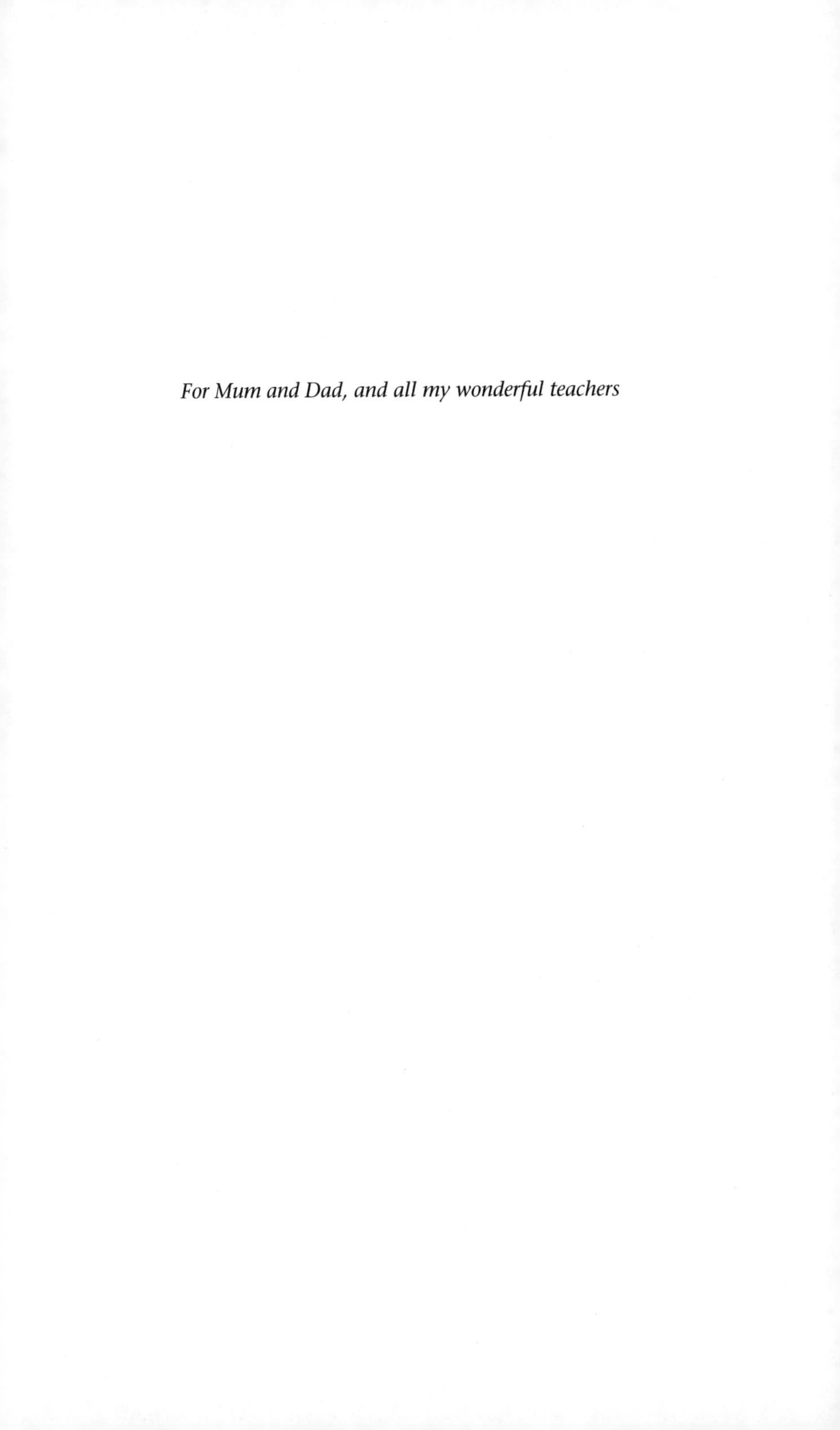

For Mum and Dad, and all my wonderful teachers

Contents

List of Illustrations

Acknowledgements

This book emerged from my first years as a lecturer in theatre and dance, beginning at the University of Mainz in Germany. Here, I would like to thank Friedemann Kreuder for his early encouragement and unconditional support of my ideas for teaching and curriculum development. Several ideas for this project emerged in those early days from our theatre visits, conversations, research seminars and, last but not least, a final conference when I was already in the United Kingdom titled "Take Up the Bodies! – Theatralität und Schrift/Kultur, 1968–2008" held at the University of Mainz in July 2008.

At the University of Aberystwyth in Wales, the project took on further shape and slowly evolved into the current book under the continued guidance from my research mentor and dear friend Heike Roms who helped me transition between the German and UK educational systems as I developed the module "The Body in 20th Century Theatre and Dance" as a lecture series and performance workshop team-taught with my other wonderful colleague in dance Margaret Ames. Her practice research with Cyrff Ystwyth Dance Company became invaluable for my deepened understanding of the dancing body in performance, and its connection to self and creativity was further spurred by a summer workshop I took with Anne Halprin in California in 2009. In the initial proposal phase, several other friends and colleagues at Aberystwyth helped to get the book project on its feet. I would like to thank Adrian Kear, Carl Lavery, Mike Pearson and Andrew Filmer for their feedback and time to discuss my early ideas for this book. Long-standing support also came from my research mentors Christopher Balme and Martin Puchner, who both provided their insight and invaluable experience to help me keep steady on my journey as an early career researcher between different countries and languages.

Several archives and institutions have provided further guidance and resource materials along the way. Here I would like to thank Richard Gough and the Centre for Performance Research for their assistance and access to invaluable resource materials, especially their vast collection of performance videos and documentation, as well as Paul

Allain and the British Grotowski Project at University of Kent. I would also like to thank Erika Fischer-Lichte and Gabriele Brandstetter at the Interweaving Performance Cultures research centre in Berlin. A generous research fellowship granted me an annual leave from 2011 to 2012 to work especially on the last section of this book, but also to access archival materials at the Freie Universität Berlin.

My thanks extend to the editorial team at Palgrave, especially Lucinda Knight and Clarissa Sutherland as well as all photographers, theatre and dance companies who provided permission to use their photographs during the last weeks. Especially I would like to thank Anett Schubotz and the Bertolt Brecht Archive Berlin, Karolina Wycisk at the Grotowski Institute Wrocław, as well as Lynn Wichern at Merce Cunningham Trust. A special thanks goes to Nan Melville, Bernd Uhlig, Herman Sorgeloos, Bettina Stöß, Alastair Muir and Jackie Guy for their photographs of Martha Graham Dance Company and Alvin Ailey American Dance Theatre, Anne Teresa De Keersmaeker, Sasha Waltz & Guests, as well as Wuppertal Tanztheater, National Theatre and Sadler's Wells.

This book could not have been written without the continuous inspiration from all my students at the Universities of Mainz, Aberystwyth and Surrey – thank you for taking an interest in the body with me and sharing all your lovely thoughts and performances as a result! You have been absolutely wonderful, and I hope you will keep dancing into your old age. I also thank Vijay Khuttan for first introducing me to the Buddhist teachings and being a true soulmate over those last years, as well as the London Shambhala Centre in Clapham – their introduction to Shambhala arts workshops and Chögyam Trungpa's *True Perception. The Path of Dharma Art* (1994) has been truly revelatory.

These are times of change for higher education in the United Kingdom, and I want to thank my colleagues Andy Lavender and Laura Cull for their continuous support of dance at the University of Surrey over the past two years. As corporatization and university league table rankings put the arts under pressure, we often struggle to demonstrate the value of dance and theatre in a world that appears to more and more be dominated by corporate finance and its dogmatic rules. However, as the book hopes to assert, there is value for us to examine the sometimes rather invisible outcomes of performance research as its merits point us towards a more sustainable, peaceful future and to remind ourselves to "put the body on the line" if needs be.

Sabine Sörgel, March 2015

Preface

Dance and the Body in Western Theatre since 1948

The mid to late twentieth century has been widely regarded as the century of the body, when philosophers, cultural critics, sociologists and theatre historians spent inordinate amounts of time and energy locating, dissecting and celebrating the body. While the body appears in almost all cultural discourses, it is nowhere as visible, as exposed as in dance, and yet dance is not considered in most theatre histories at all. In this book I seek to capture this obsession with the dancing body post 1948 where it is most evident: in a number of significant stage performances of the Western canon. The book examines key theatre and dance practitioners from Antonin Artaud and Bertolt Brecht, Martha Graham, Jerzy Grotowski and Peter Brook, to Pina Bausch, Anne Teresa de Keersmaeker and Akram Khan among others to demonstrate what can be argued is a major shift towards dance and somatic practice in Western theatre today.

By initiating the little known history of dance in post-1948 Western theatre, I first of all seek to unravel the hidden politics and sociocultural dynamics of the body in the Western imagination. Dance becomes the lens through which perceptions of the body need to be reconfigured in the context of an emerging human rights culture and transnational politics after the Second World War. More than simply offer a canonical survey of major Western performances from continental Europe, Great Britain, and the United States, the book presents new perspectives on Western theatre by placing dance at the centre of competing ideological battles over democracy, decolonization and world citizenship during the Cold War era up to the present moment. A major trajectory of the book will be to examine how the body in performance responds to political challenge and change post 1948, as for example such historical events as the 1968 countercultural revolution and Vietnam War, the fall of the Berlin Wall in 1989 and contemporary consumer society, globalization and the crisis of late capitalism post 9/11 into our present.

The book covers a selection of canonical directors and choreographers, all of whom infused their theatre with experiential impulses from the body. Despite their diverging training techniques and modes of rehearsal, all of them resort to the resurrection of the body as a political force to be counted on. By interlocking the perspectives of dance and theatre in these works, we see how studying dance allows us to understand the connection between distinct movement practices and changing cultural dynamics in performance. Discourses in dance shaped the sociopolitical discourses of the body at their time while also reflecting upon political questions such as the redefinition of humanism post 1948, which prepared for the newly emerging cosmopolitanism and human rights culture of today.

The chapter divisions are largely based on a lecture series for an undergraduate module called "The Body in 20th Century Theatre and Dance" held at the Universities of Mainz, Aberystwyth and Surrey over the past eight years, which introduced students to key theoretical concepts in phenomenology, kinaesthetic awareness, cognitive science, imaginal psychology and cultural studies. Placing the body at the centre of this endeavour, the book allows students an easy access point from which to undertake individual further studies of corporeality in their own performance practice. Each chapter focuses on at least one major critical concept for analysis and juxtaposes up to three indicative performances for this suggested shift towards dance. The book uses online documentation of live works as opposed to dramatic texts to familiarize you with key issues and theories of and on the body in performance. To do this, basic readings in phenomenology, neuroscience and philosophy are introduced to give you major theoretical concepts for performance analysis such as embodiment, ritual and cultural identity, archetype and the collective unconscious throughout the individual chapters. Illustrations and further suggestions for reading and performance work available online and on DVDs facilitate your own engagement and research on the topic. This didactic approach provides you with an in-depth analysis of the genealogy of the body in twentieth-century theatre and dance, while at the same time delivering a canonical overview and further reference for key twentieth-century theatre directors and dance choreographers up to the present. As such the book serves as an accessible introduction to new critical approaches in performance historiography as well as offering a practice-informed investigation of corporeality between theatre and dance. Most of the discussed works are either commercially available on DVD or freely accessible online for you to undertake further study of the theoretical aspects discussed based on the study questions provided at the end of each section. Taken together, these multiple perspectives hope to offer a wide critical framework to demonstrate how dance entered twentieth-century theatre historiography and how it continues to influence our thinking about the body today.

1 The Body, Dance and Phenomenology

Dance and the moving body: From breath to consciousness

One of the major objectives of this book is to look at dance and examine how it has changed images of the body and self throughout the twentieth century and its theatre performances. Movement is in many ways our first bodily encounter of the world, before we start to develop further awareness and language skills to communicate with other people. As Sondra Fraleigh asserts, "[D]ance founds the meaning that words name" (1987, p. 73). Most of our experiences of the world are thus based in movement, and our "sense-making originates in species-specific kinetic understandings emanating from a common body of movement" (Sheets-Johnstone, 2009, p. 15). As Maxine Sheets-Johnstone further explains, to improvise a dance is interestingly our most immediate response to existing in the world:

> To say that in improvising, I am in the process of creating the dance out of the possibilities which are mine at any moment of the dance is to say that I am exploring the world in movement; that is, at the same time that I am moving, I am taking into account the world as it exists for me here and now in this ongoing, ever-expanding present. As one might wonder about the world in words, I am wondering the world directly, in movement. (2009, p. 31)

In a sense, this approach towards movement in dance improvisation is assertive of our individual creativity as human beings, who experience the world through movement. Dance, as we will see, choreographs experience and produces knowledge, which sometimes even spurs social movements such as in some of the cases explored in this book. Yet, as much as we forget about our bodies in everyday life, we also tend to forget and not see the dance that unfolds in every little move that we make.

Life begins with the pulsing heart and a scream that inhales oxygen into our lungs, as we take our first breath, and pumps it through our veins into the brain. From then on we start to perceive the world and distinguish between light and shade, colours, shapes and forms to reveal ever more clear images of the world as we slowly begin to make sense. A baby responds to the voice as it hears sounds inside the womb; a little hand grasping for your finger relates touch to a pleasurable feeling, an instinctive reflex, seeking protection perhaps, as wide eyes smile back at you in astonishment of this wonder: what does it all mean? Emotion plays out in a glance and a smile that touches you at the core, often described as a warm feeling rising up from the belly, before it is registered by the brain as something initially felt before worded: joy.

Antonio Damasio, a renowned neuroscientist whose research investigates the relation between brain function and consciousness, refers to the body as the theatre of our emotions (2000, p. 4). He believes that emotion is the evolutionary foundation from which human consciousness was developed and employs the theatrical metaphor to explain how "feelings perform their ultimate and longer-lasting effects in the theatre of the conscious mind" (2000, p. 37). As natural-born performers, we do of course know about this, since we constantly negotiate our own emotional worlds with the social roles we play from day to day as we grow up. Our acting careers start early on in our life, when we begin to perform our self on a daily basis. As human beings, we act in response to our emotions as well as the natural and sociocultural environment we are born into. And yet, before the acting comes the dance, which is the primary movement of breath in our lungs, the inner pulse of life lived and our first encounter with time and rhythm.

Damasio hence identifies three levels of self to demonstrate traces of our evolutionary development located within our bodies' emotional landscape. He calls the first level the "proto-self" or "nonconscious forerunner", while "core self" and "autobiographical self", the second and third levels, both refer to the "conscious protagonists" of our mind (2000, p. 22). Basically, Damasio argues that the self as a notion originated as the backdrop upon which "the feeling of emotion [first became] known to the organism having the emotion" (2000, p. 8). As a matter of fact, we often feel before we know and refer to such wordless premonition of knowledge as our intuition or sixth sense.

Damasio explains how this drama of human consciousness and existence unfolds neurophysiologically:

> You know you exist because the narrative exhibits you as protagonist in the act of knowing. You rise above the sea level of knowing, transiently but incessantly, as a felt core of self, renewed again and again, thanks to anything that comes from outside the brain into its sensory machinery or anything that comes from the brain's memory stores toward sensory, motor, or autonomic recall. (2000, p. 172)

The fact that consciousness is born, when we first perceive the outside world in images of objects, furthermore adheres to a dramaturgy which, again, dance and theatre students know particularly well. As Damasio outlines the structural element of our so-called movies-in-the-brain:

> This account is a simple narrative without words. It does have characters (the organism, the object). It unfolds in time. And it has a beginning, a middle, and an end. The beginning corresponds to the initial state of the organism. The middle is the arrival of the object. The end is made up of reactions that result in a modified state of the organism. (2000, p. 169)

Damasio claims that it is due to core consciousness that we instantly construct such images on the basis of neural patterning as an evolutionary strategy of survival (2000, pp. 37, 126). Emotions are key in this process, and according to Damasio's hypothesis, they coincide with core consciousness (2000, pp. 37, 100, 169).

As human beings, we thus share a biological core of six primary emotions (happiness, sadness, fear, anger, surprise and disgust), as already outlined by Paul Ekman (*1934) in the 1970s, yet we also complicate matters in the way that so-called background emotions are far more diverse and individual (Damasio, 2000, pp. 50–51). Emotions and feelings play out along a three-level continuum which starts from an initial, often non-conscious state of emotion towards a state of feeling then made conscious (2000, p. 37). Thoughts and actions in our mind therefore evolve from a continuous loop of emotion which triggers feeling to result in yet another emotion to create a new feeling and so on (2000, p. 43).

Phenomenology and kinaesthetic awareness

The proposed methodology for our study takes a fresh look at phenomenology for its radical critique of Western rationalism and its ideological premises and conceptualizations. Phenomenology in dance studies has thus far largely been used as a descriptive hermeneutics for movement analysis. While this book follows this tradition to a certain extent, its major challenge is to unveil the hidden politics of a radical phenomenology of life and creative potential in the wake of the philosophical writings of Michel Henry (1922–2002) and Bernhard Waldenfels (*1934). It is argued that phenomenology and dance allow us to rethink the world and its politics at any time by transcending the limited notion of Western anthropocentrism by focusing on our felt response to life and ecology. Suggesting that the self is not so much a scientific but felt subjectivity, a phenomenology of life questions the hegemony of the Western scientific model grounded in seventeenth-century models of geometry and materialism. Rather, in and through dance we assert the fact that our subjectivity is experienced as the immanence of life affecting human existence at the core of felt experience. It is by creatively affirming the felt quality of life that the dancer expresses freedom as the outward transcendence of self and individuality – the basic condition for freedom and solidarity in a democratic society.

Phenomenology, as a strand within Western philosophy, is often referred to as an archaeology of the mind, because it traces the different layers of our evolving consciousness which is itself not easy to define as we have seen, but can be described as the mind's underlying structural matrix upon which experience is inscribed (Fellmann, 2006, pp. 38–40). To look at consciousness as a pre-given matrix allows us to see that consciousness is the necessary precondition for us to not only have experiences in the first place but also recall and reflect upon such experiences to articulate them in more sophisticated ways, such as the evolution of language to name our experiences or to alter and adapt simple movements that we have once learnt into more challenging ones. Human consciousness is thus based in our several kinaesthetic senses which allow us to see, touch, smell, hear, move and taste. With Sondra Fraleigh we may say that dance improvisation is indeed the lived expression of our "pure consciousness" and kinaesthetic awareness of sensually being in space. She explains,

> As the dance is fully realized, it ceases to be an object of consciousness; it dissolves in perfected action. To understand the dancer as the

> dance is to understand a point of unification, which is a state of being when the dance is lived not as an object but as a pure consciousness. (1987, p. 40)

Hence, a phenomenological approach starts by interrogating the origin of sense perception so that we can describe how meaning is created in dance by using the body's sensual apparatus. In dance, self-awareness is often at one with our movement – body and mind are not separated, but one.

As human beings, our bodies are always positioned in relation to the world, and a central phenomenological concept to distinguish human experience by this fact is intentionality (Fellmann, 2006, p. 57). Intentionality refers to our movement-based engagement with the objects of the world as sense-making is characterized by our specific intentions towards engaging with the environment. The body serves as our spatial index according to which our experience of any given situation is measured. Felt intuition and emotional impulse initiate this process as they underlie the intention of any given action. More importantly, intentionality evokes our sense of space as we consider and assess our environment according to objects and phenomena within our reach and view or even by our smell.

While intentionality is directed towards objects outside our conscious awareness, our felt intuition that forms the conscious awareness is pre-given to experience, and Henri Bergson (1859–1941) was perhaps the first philosopher who pointed towards this passivity of consciousness in relation to our feeling-based intentions towards the world (Fellmann, 2006, p. 124). Human experience hence mediates in relation to the perceived sensual data or givens of the environment and does not so much rely on rational or subjective principles but an interior impulse to move or act. Self-consciousness is thus derived from our affective responses to environmental or interpersonal triggers. This affective impulse is often referred to as the spiritual energy of life itself and finds many parallel conceptualizations and healing attributes in non-Western cultures such as Chi in China, Reiki in Japan, or Ashé among the Yoruba in Nigeria, as well as Kundalini in India. In Kundalini yoga, for example, life energy is experienced as a moving force coiled at the bottom of our spine where it instigates all our responsive engagement with the environment as it moves upwards through the different energy centres known as chakras. Our pelvis, belly, solar plexus, throat and third eye (the spot between the eyebrows leading into the crown of the head) thus carry specific levels of energy as the expression of our creativity and potential in life (see Kumar and Larsen, 2004; Zeltzer, 2011). While this energy can be experienced as predominantly sexual and procreative, it is more expansive than that as it ultimately surpasses our ego conception and concern for the self, akin to the experience we may have in deep meditation, sexual union and also dance. Somatically, if we follow this energy up the spine to our brain, we can see how the human skeleton embodies traces of our evolution – from water to the four-footed stand of the animal to our upright standing position – as continued shifts in balance overcoming gravity – phases each human still goes through within the first year of their life (Keleman, 1985, p. 25).

In that sense, our birth figures as a somewhat traumatic experience. Thrown into the world, we gasp for air and feel ourselves in motion, continuously learning from suffering as the world forthwith evolves around us more than we actually control it. Michel Henry's phenomenology of life refers to such emotional responding as "pathos" (2002), an intense suffering or pain as we psychologically depart from the curled creature swimming happily sheltered in the womb to individuality and separation from our mothers first but further on entering the cycle of change and impermanence of our lived reality. Suffering is therefore often considered as the quintessential experience of human existence as described in world religions ranging from Christianity to Buddhism as well as modern philosophy or even the history of Western drama, where pathos – a suffering from fate – marked the archetypal heroes of Greek tragedy and initiated audiences into a powerful recognition of their moral sensibility referred to as catharsis or ritualistic cleansing (Aristotle, 1996 [335 BCE]). Religion, philosophy and psychology have long since marvelled at the origin of our feeling-toned response to the world and located core consciousness or intuition not so much in the human brain but the soul. The soul, however, is a troubled concept today as we can neither scientifically measure its scale nor locate it anatomically, leading many people to doubt its existence. And yet, philosophers and artists persistently cherish the soul as the source of our initial response to music, love or nature. It is the feeling-toned soul rather than the mind that helps us to think what we feel, and yet we fail to measure it adequately in mathematical scales or words. The soul thus refers to the yet-unresolved mystery of life and existence. It is the invisible key to our self as experienced in feeling.

Now, before you continue reading this book, take a minute and experience your own body: how do you feel? Is there any particular part of your body that you notice and why? After you woke up this morning, was there anything you did to your body to make it look the way it does just now? Is your body a he or a she – and how do you know? Do you identify with your body – is it you? Take a few minutes and consider your answers and note how we often feel our body one way from the inside, while the outside appearance may tell us yet another story. We usually take our body for granted, and interestingly enough we often tend to almost forget about the body unless it starts to hurt and makes us feel unwell. Our personal experience of the body is thus shaped by an inside feeling-toned perception that directly relates to the outside environment and other people.

As this experiment shows, we notice our body most severely when we feel pain, but the body also allows for the feeling of great pleasure and exhilaration, as in orgasm. Philosopher Jean-Luc Marion (*1946) argues that such intense feeling saturates experience to the extent that the body feels itself from the inside, while paradoxically this feeling is given from elsewhere, the lover or an accident, for example (see Marion, 2002). This is so because such intense feelings are not only anatomical but also imagined in a complex working of body–mind continuum, and memory, pain and pleasure involve all three levels of our proto-self, core self and autobiographical self. The body in these instances is also referred to as "flesh" in order to account for the vulnerability of our embodied existence, as well as the receiving openness our bodies allow for when lived existence is seen as a metaphysical gift (see Marion, 2002). Birth and death, and hopefully love, are such great gifts beyond our control as we await the event of their coming into being. These events play a major role in defining human existence on the levels of proto-self, core self and autobiographical self and have often been responded to and celebrated in dance. Although we do invest a whole lot of feeling in our experience of pleasure and pain, we have to notice that these are not emotions in the strict neurophysiological sense, but events or givens. The feeling of pain affiliated with death will be particularly interesting when we turn to our case studies in the following chapters of this book, as many a theatre dance has evolved around this theme between the two world wars of the twentieth century.

Body–mind in Western philosophy

Taking a phenomenological perspective on feeling and emotion as embodied experiences of mind and consciousness, it appears quite strange that Western philosophy from the Greeks up to the present has perceived the body in terms of a subject/object dichotomy. Performance artists in the 1960s rebelled against this flawed separation which is still very prevalent in Western capitalist societies. Later on, we consider the political implications of the artists' resistance in order to demonstrate how their increased interest in the body initiates an aesthetic return towards dance as a privileged paradigm for counter-knowledge formation today. Not only does this shift impact the formal aspects of theatre work that increasingly looks and feels like dance but we will discover how the dancing body also redefines the relationship of the individual performer in relation to the ensemble and audience.

However, before we can understand how this shift towards dance occurred in the mid-twentieth century, it is important to review some of the history behind the old and lasting prejudices against the body. Philosophers traditionally saw it as the natural body, physiological body, and its cultural counterpart. Since the seventeenth century, this mode of thinking privileged the mind as a separate spiritual entity in the wake of René Descartes's (1596–1650) Latin "cogito" as "thinking I", somewhat independent and more importantly in control of the body's more carnal activities (eating, digestion, sex, etc.). Bodily secretions and carnal pleasures were considered as a sign of human weakness, whereas the mind became the powerhouse and centre of control.

Along those lines, we find a philosophic tendency which separates thought processes from our emotional responses, although this is hardly the case as Damasio's more recent findings in neuroscience show. However, following this tradition of neglect, we often mistrust our emotions and privilege the rational as the superior response. In that sense, the mind was regarded as active and in rational control of the emotional and therefore passive and weak body. While the body was a natural given, the mind could be culturally formed and enlightened and thus influence and shape the body accordingly. The problem with the prevalent body–mind dualism in Western philosophy is not only that it ignored the interdependency of body–mind but more importantly that it objectified the body, which is in fact never an object but subject to our world. As anthropologist

Thomas J. Csordas describes this dilemma: "Objectification is the product of reflective, ideological knowledge, whether it be in the form of colonial Christianity, biological science, or consumer culture" (1994, p. 7).

Such objectification of the body has many faces. Look at yourself in the mirror, for example, and instantly you start to separate your body from an inner experience of self into an outward projection or self-image. French philosopher Jacques Lacan (1901–1981) refers to this level as mirror stage, when a child first starts to think of herself as independent from her mother (2006, pp. 75–81). This idea of the mirror image is still very prevalent in our contemporary media culture, from magazines and commercials to TV, film and Facebook. Without us even noticing, we constantly live up to those images and identities which we create and surround ourselves with. Likewise, in our interactions with other people, their look may turn us into an object of their gaze. Women, for example, may be objectified as stylized sex symbols, such as pop icons Shakira or Beyoncé, despite their assertive agency in producing their commercialized celebrity performances. Because these mediatized images are everywhere today, we are likely to build our identities based on the outside recognition of ourselves as objectified products with the fashionable haircut and designer clothes at hand rather than developing trust in our inner emotional experience. More often than we perhaps realize, many of us live up to those images of other bodies projected by the mirror and other media, instead of listening to our intuition and felt response to find our original source for creative expression.

If we look into the history of the self in Western society, we can thus find an illustrious number of quotes that have tried to define our existence. Guess who may have said the following:

"I think, therefore I am."
"I shop therefore I am."
"The mind is a muscle."

Take a few minutes and consider your answers. What is the shift in emphasis, and what are you for today? To conclude, Western philosophies of body–mind dualism refer to a mode of thinking where our notion of self and identity is determined by the interplay of emotion, consciousness and language. From the seventeenth-century philosopher of the enlightenment René Descartes's cogito ("I think, therefore

I am"), to late capitalism ("I shop therefore I am") and postmodern dancer Yvonne Rainer ("The mind is a muscle") body–mind continues to shape our notion of identity today.

Towards analysis: A phenomenological perspective

As a methodology for performance analysis, phenomenology starts from the premise that our initial sense perception does not distinguish between experience and judgement so that theory and practice are at one. A phenomenologist seeks to relate to the world via returning to such immediate perception which simply means that one starts to account for an experience as first inwardly felt and given to the senses. One way to do this easily is via an exercise in kinaesthetic awareness. Take off your shoes and socks, for example, then close your eyes and notice your breathing pattern. Where do your feet touch the ground? Wriggle your toes and shift balance. Listen to the sounds in the room. How does that make you feel? Do any inner images occur? What is your sense of the immediate space or kinesphere that surrounds you? It is often hard to describe the meaning of a dance movement or step with words as we often lack the proper concept or name for it unless we are well versed in ballet vocabulary or notation, which most theatre audiences are certainly not. Why would they still enjoy watching a dance? After all, what does it mean to watch someone wriggling their toes with eyes closed? We may not know, and still find it enjoyable or amusing to observe. The phenomenologist's answer would be that we have an intuited emotional response that affects us immediately as we inwardly dance along. Some dances may make us feel happy while others may appear boring, have a sad or even aggressive tone. It is the feeling-toned impact that matters in dance and phenomenology, as has also been proven by the more recent findings of neuroscience referred to before.

The fact that we dance along while watching has therefore been conceptualized as what is called kinaesthetic empathy. This basically means that we imitate more or less all movements that we see by rehearsing them in the brain (see Foster, 2011; Reynolds and Reason, 2012). Hence, someone taking of her shoes and wriggling the toes may have us wonder about what it would feel like to do the same, as your own feet are probably squeezed into those tight heels to match your beautiful evening dress. So even if we were never to become professional dancers ourselves, the more dances we watch and the more aware of movement we become, the better experts in judging dance we will be, and that is simply according to how our brain works through and with movement any single second of our lives. To watch a dance is therefore the first step for us to learn about new movements, as our life expands with each breath that we take. As everybody already dances the minute they are born, dance, on its most fundamental level, encapsulates our energetic engagement with the moving world around us each day of our lives. Note that this is also the way that many dance classes are organized, as we learn either by observing and imitating our teacher, or working with movement that emerges from an inwardly felt energetic impulse.

While our focus in phenomenology is on experience and movement, language is still a powerful tool to communicate and share our felt experiences with other people. Thus, we come up with words for our felt sensations, such as headache, toothache, chill, etc., and thereby learn to communicate our emotional world to others. While such intense feelings as heartache may vary significantly from one person to another – as many other of our more complex inter-human emotional relationships – words are often still our best bet to make us heard and receive help. Although language hardly gives us an accurate account of subjective experience, it is often the easiest and most efficient way to communicate. Language in everyday life is therefore used as if it provided a universally true representation of our emotional states, even though that is not necessarily the case.

Logocentrism refers to this privileging of the word as a conveyor of truth, as is written in the bible: "In the beginning was the word [= logos]" (John 1:1). However, note that logos, as many other Greek words, does have several more meanings and interestingly enough could also mean reason or spirit. Hence, the word as logos is in fact body–mind, although Western logocentrism increasingly separated the word from the body's relation to spirit and breath. As Western societies departed from their religious beliefs in the process of modernization, words became increasingly devoid of spirit and thus established language as a tool for communication. The word hence suffers from the same objectification as the body, for as soon as we fix meaning to the object, any room for creativity is stifled. However, as we can see in the study of poetry, language does have the power to re-enchant words with their own spirit, and so does dance with respect to the body, when meaning is again opened up to subjective feeling and interpretation.

Language serves as a powerful mediator between experience and expression, but it is never the exact same as our inner experience of the world, nor its outside objects despite the fact that we often use it that way in everyday life. Hence, we can think of language in parallel to the body as it too creates our theatre of emotion, yet via sounded and written words rather than movement vocabulary. In any case, neither words nor movement allow for any claims as to the truth of the objects that we encounter in the form of images in our mind or the existence of a reality outside our own imagination of it. And yet, experientially we would be able to claim as truthful that which is in accord with our felt experience as we perceive ourselves deeply connected to the outside world.

Similar to our ignorance of the complex functioning of the body in everyday life, we also ignore the complexity of language and writing as we take words for objective truth and thus establish social categories and norms. Csordas, in his quote above, referred to such normative use of language as ideological, because it creates whole belief systems around it. Philosopher Michel Foucault (1926–1984) analysed the relationship between language and power arguing that words, by naming and representing the world, create the illusion of truth. While such truth is based on convention and agreement on words referencing certain objects and relationships between people in society, language establishes what Foucault has called "discourse", meaning a whole set of societal beliefs and standards. In his important works, *The Order of Things, The Archaeology of Knowledge, Discipline and Punish* as well as *The History of Sexuality*, Foucault demonstrated that the analysis of language (= discourse in French) helps us understand the institutionalized patterns of power in society. For example, sexually frustrated women in the nineteenth century were treated for hysteria during a time before the women's and sexual liberation movement. Western colonialism in the sixteenth and seventeenth centuries rationalized slavery by categorizing indigenous peoples as uncivilized due to their different colour of skin, foreign customs, religious beliefs, dance forms and languages. Colonialism as a racist discourse manifested in travel writings and novels of the period, thus objectified foreign bodies to exploit their labour force during the Atlantic slave trade. And there are many more examples, for example, young women suffering from anorexia due to an abusive fetishization of slimness in the media, etc.

Language thus codifies and fixes meaning as if it was set in stone and thereby serves human civilization as a powerful tool to organize communication, build national communities and political empires, as well as to gather and disseminate knowledge. We identify with people who speak our own language, because not only do we share the same words but most often we also have similar social structures, historical memories, etc. Hence, language has a very strong tradition as the basis of cultural knowledge in Western societies, and we will have to analyse language and writing when we consider the body in twentieth-century theatre, although our main interest is in dance as an alternative way of experiencing and knowing via movement.

To examine the dancing body from a phenomenological perspective hence acknowledges the body's mediating function in the birth of our consciousness by reflecting that we cannot know beforehand what is immediately experienced as such. Sondra Fraleigh explains,

> The self known in dance is indeed a performing self and is at its best as it moves toward such freedom. The self known in dance moves beyond the limits of our mental cogito. We dance to become acquainted with that which cannot be known by any other means – to find out what can be known through the body as mental, physical, spiritual whole. (1987, p. 26)

When we analyse dance, Fraleigh's phenomenological approach appears particularly useful since dance does not provide the performer with a written dramatic text to start from. Although we may find something similar to the dramatic concepts of role and character in romantic ballets like *Swan Lake* or *Giselle,* modern dance often confronts us with a repertoire of movements developed by the dancer and choreographer to convey a certain emotion, something more abstract and yet very close to our intuition and core consciousness of felt self. Each dance thus presents an expression of how we align our bodies with a concept of self embodied by the dance.

However, dance performers are usually trained in a certain movement or dance vocabulary – ballet, modern, contemporary, popular, standard or folk dance – to enable them to perform a specific choreography. Depending on the dance at hand, dance scholar Susan Foster therefore suggests that we also need to analyse the dancing body as a "body of ideas" (1997, pp. 235–257) and interrogate specific cultural and aesthetic contexts for each dance we examine. She introduces the term "corporeality" to reflect on the fact that many of our understandings of the dancing body are shaped by society and discourse (see Foster, 1995). Dance in Europe, for example, will have a different history, style and aesthetic than dance from South Asia or the African continent, because of different musical traditions and dance forms. If we consider romantic ballet, for example, we can look at the ballerina as introducing a specific type of female beauty that is delicate, dancing on her toes, light and airy and as such very different from the earthbound expressiveness of barefoot modern dance thereafter. However, since the early explorers' expeditions of the sixteenth- and seventeenth-centuries' dance forms have also travelled and mutually informed each other and while some dances are examples of cultural diversity, other dance forms have blended into a global movement repertoire, and such classical techniques as ballet and South Asian Kathak and Bharatanatyam are meanwhile taught across cultures and countries (see Katrak, 2011; Soneji, 2010).

In the following analyses of twentieth-century theatre and dance performances we will consider the relationship between embodied experience, language and dance as well as introduce several important theories and discourses surrounding the moving bodies on stage at their time. Thereby we will see how we have to shift focus onto the dancing body – what and how it means – depending on the different approaches taken by each director and choreographer examined in the book. Experiencing the body is crucial in all the chosen works of twentieth-century theatre directors and dance choreographers examined here, and they present an indicative survey of how twentieth-century dance practices have changed the way we look at the body today. Although this can hardly be conclusive considering the many performances not mentioned here, the following chapters seek to challenge your perception of the body on the Western stage and hope to encourage your own research on the topic.

Study Questions:

1. What is consciousness?
2. What is the relationship between movement and feeling?
3. Consider the meaning of emotion – how does it shape our sense of self?
4. When would you say that you first started to dance?
5. How can we use phenomenology to analyse dance?

2 Writing Dance into Theatre

Antonin Artaud's Affective Athleticism

In the depth of time: Artaud's poetics of affect and the writing of dance into theatre

Antonin Artaud was born in 1896 and suffered from childhood illnesses caused by an early attack of meningitis at the age of only four from which he never fully recovered. The young Artaud subsequently developed a stammer and put up with severe headaches for all his life. As a teenager, he was treated for depression for the first time, and his doctors prescribed opium which caused an early addiction in the adolescent. Pain became Artaud's lifelong companion, and his poetic writings mirror this experience (see Barber, 1993). He became interested in Surrealism, an art movement of the early twentieth century in France which concerned itself with the impact of the subconscious and its evocation of inner images directly linked to the analysis of dreams introduced by Sigmund Freud (1856–1939). Artaud became increasingly ill and was successively held in different mental institutions in Northern France throughout his life. This is the period during which Artaud wrote *The Theatre and Its Double*, and the alternating spells of schizophrenia and lucidity may explain some of the erratic style of writing. In 1943 Artaud was transferred to the infamous clinic at Rodez where he was treated with electroshock therapy. Artaud continued his writing during this period, and there are several self-portraits and drawings which he produced during this time of extreme psycho-physical torment (see Grossman, 2008). He also finished his *Travel to the Land of the Tarahumaras* (1945) – an account of his travels to Mexico. In 1946 he was released from the mental hospital and stayed for another year at a rest home at Ivry, on the outskirts of Paris. He was very weak at that time and looked like a shadow of himself in the photographs that still exist from this period (see Franzke and Trujillo, 2006). The last document that we have is a radio broadcast called *To Have Done with the Judgement of God* which he had been commissioned for in 1947/48. While the broadcast was never transmitted at its time, as it was considered too obscene, it is now regarded as the closest example of the theatre of cruelty in performance. At this time, Artaud was also diagnosed with terminal cancer, and he died on the 4 March 1948 (see Barber, 1993).

When we read Artaud, students in my seminars often ask why they have to study the writings of a lunatic, and that is indeed a very good question to pursue. I especially enjoy hearing the word "lunatic" for Artaud, because it brings together the schizophrenic state of mind under the influence of the lunar cycle and is hence bound up with nature and the cosmos, both of which are crucial for Artaud's conception of a future theatre. The answer I usually give, however, is that we study him because he had such an extraordinary influence on the generation that followed next, not only artists but also philosophers and cultural critics such as Gilles Deleuze (1925–1995), Jaques Derrida (1930–2004) or Susan Sontag (1933–2004). More recently, Artaud is now also flagged up as a proto-fascist. While the majority of twentieth-century critics tend to read Artaud's dark poetics as a felt response to his life of severe pain and suffering, more recent interpretations look at the destructive rhetoric of his work in relation to rising fascist sentiments of the time (see Jannarone, 2010). Indeed, I think that the controversy surrounding Artaud continues to provoke interest precisely because his poetry points a finger at uncomfortable truths about the human psyche. Artaud's writing is out of control and presents nightmarish visions of death and destruction very close to the reality of the two world wars which marked the twentieth century. Each study of his work needs to carefully examine this lurking fascist underside of his writing in its historical context, because it is part of human nature whether we like it or not.

Artaud's writing and schizophrenia continue to present a paradox to the critic, because his dense and destructive imagery confronts the reader with the darker side of human consciousness and awareness. Lunacy may thus take us towards death and destruction but it also highlights the creative potential of poetic language, unconscious imagery and the inner landscape. The brief account of Artaud's life shows that his biography and lyricism cannot be separated from each other as indeed Artaud's life was his art – and the schizophrenia is always apparent as a self-reflexive mode of writing. As Gilles Deleuze points out,

> For the schizophrenic, then, it is less a question of recovering meaning than of destroying the word, of conjuring up the affect, and of transforming the painful passion of the body into a triumphant action, obedience into command, always in this depth beneath the fissured surface. (Deleuze, 2004 [1969], p. 100)

To understand Artaud's aesthetic, it is important to gain an insight from reading his poetry as the writing of his life-dance into theatre, violent as it may be. The source of Artaud's poetic skills emerges from the creative impulse that struggles to account for the lived experience of schizophrenia and electroshock treatment. Artaud's schizophrenic mind is one that does not follow the principles of logic and coherent subjectivity but rather experiences the world in multifarious bodily sensations and dispersed inner images. (See Artaud, 2011.)

In a way one could argue with Damasio that Artaud's poetic mind operates largely on core-conscious impulses from a pre-subjective layer of the rational mind located in the neocortex of our brain. Language becomes no(n)-sense to the degree that it no longer adheres to codified meaning while at the same time it is freed towards its full theatrical potential as sensuous musicality. Gilles Deleuze further explains,

> The duality of the schizophrenic word has not been adequately noted: it comprises the passion-word, which explodes into wounding phonetic values, and the action-word, which welds inarticulate tonic values. These two words are developed in relation to the duality of the body, fragmented body and body without organs. They refer to two theatres, the theatre of terror or passion and the theatre of cruelty, which is by its essence active. (2004, p. 103)

The mismatch in response to the outside world thus causes a non-mimetic art of the subject's inner life. Artaud's theatre of cruelty hence refers to a mode of performance that attacks language as a mode of mimetic representation, while at the same time it produces a language true to the inner self and world of imagination.

In that sense the impact of Balinese dance theatre which Artaud first witnessed during the 1931 International Colonial Exhibition in Paris was a crucial event, because it transgressed Western forms of theatrical realism. Even though Artaud had no cultural understanding of Balinese dance, his orientalist fascination with the form consisted in its affective tonality which combined costumes, rhythm and dance movements with mask-like facial expressions unlike Western forms of dance and acting at the time. Rustom Bharucha's cross-cultural critique of orientalist theatre in the wake of Artaud's writings carefully dissects the many misunderstandings and imperialist appropriations that led to a resurgence of dance and ritual in twentieth-century Western theatre (1993). Thus, Balinese dance theatre seemed to prove to Artaud and several others in his wake that dance and theatre emerge from the body's inner images rather than creating a replica of the outside perception of worldly matter. Although culturally unspecific in his analysis, Artaud was intuitively aware that the Balinese intentionality for dance theatre emerged from a ritualistic reverence to the sacred source of life as embodied in the danced masks of Gods, Dragons and Witches. More importantly, Balinese dance, even though already framed by a colonialist gaze and becoming a marketable tourist attraction, still embodied a cosmological life force and mythic dimension which most Western theatre in its veneration of language and dramatic form no longer conveyed. Bettina Knapp, in her essay on the mythical impact in Balinese dance theatre, characterizes this relationship as follows:

> Based on symbol and mask, Balinese theater is embedded in analogy and metonymy, and as Artaud phrased it, "correspondences". Behind each object, image, line, color, gesture, and tonality, there lay a hidden yet concrete realm: chaotic but also ecstatic and sublime. Ever alluring, this "double" sphere, as incarnated on stage, held him enthralled. (1994, p. 92)

The important terms she uses here are analogy, metonymy, correspondence or double. Her study also emphasizes the impact Balinese dance had on the autonomic nervous system, whereby movement and music evoked energetic responses in the audience.

More recently, Nicola Savarese pointed out how important Artaud's interpretation of Balinese dance theatre has become from our contemporary perspective and especially with regards to considering dance in theatre (2001, pp. 70–72). According to Savarese's reasoning here, dance serves as life's double in its non-mimetic phenomenological impact on theatre audiences by evoking a felt-kinaesthetic response. The sophistication of Balinese dance theatre is thus based in a classical form evolved over centuries. As Savarese comments,

> Like all highly disciplined actors who within highly codified forms, that is, fixed, choreographed scores, the Balinese actor-dancers make use of the entire gamut of their pre-expressive possibilities and are even able to produce, methodically – one could also say "mathematically" or "metaphysically" – a state of grace in the spectator. (2001, p. 72)

While we will return to the idea of the "state of grace" in the next chapter looking at Jerzy Grotowski's notion of holy theatre, note at this point how Savarese acknowledges the affective impact of dance by saying that because of its "pre-expressive possibilities" dance allows for a new becoming of stage language.

Not only was Artaud interested in Balinese dance theatre, but he also travelled to Mexico and investigated indigenous Mexican culture for similar reasons. He was working on a play called *The Conquest of Mexico* (1933) and was interested in the Maya as a living example of theatre of cruelty in performance. In Mexico, Artaud joined the Tarahumaras, an indigenous Mexican tribe, and sought to take part in their peyote rite. He hoped to get insights into the tribe's drug-induced ritual performances and sought to understand how they make use of incantation and animism in order to communicate with a higher spiritual force so as to gain a deeper understanding of life. Again, we see how Artaud was fascinated by the idea of a spiritual essence underlying the double-nature of our experience. However, the whole journey was problematic because of Artaud's own health problems and drug abuse. Large parts of his travel writings read, therefore, rather hallucinatory and have nothing to do with an understanding of the Tarahumara culture, but everything to do with Artaud's suffering (see Bharucha, 1993, p. 16). And yet again, there are some points that we find in Artaud's concept of a theatre of cruelty that emerged from the experience. As Luis O. Arata explains,

> Among the Tarahumara, and for the first time, Artaud would be an active participant in the drama he sought. He wished to be moved

> and transformed by this new experience, purified like an alchemist in quest of the philosopher's stone. Artaud became a spectator clinging to a repressed reality, confronting the very type of drama he had failed to create and which now he could hardly comprehend. (1994, p. 83)

Important is thus the notion of active participation in the ritualistic context, something that Artaud wanted to resurrect for Western theatre experience as well. Only if the spectator was to be transformed by his or her experience in the theatre could the event be perceived as cruel in Artaud's own understanding of the term. Performance as ritual hence becomes a revelation which changes our perception of ourselves as well as the world. Arata continues to explain,

> Ritual theater tries to reach beyond the context of the performance. It seeks to overflow its own boundaries and communicate with something beyond itself. If there is a message in ritual theater, it is one that would be received through the performance rather than conveyed by it. (1994, p. 86)

Artaud's theatre of cruelty thereby flags up theatre's transformative potential and creativity. Music, colours, movement and sound are at the heart of the Artaudian project of a theatre that is truly inventive and original. Such a theatre is close to dance, drawing from spiritual sources, inner affective experience and suggestion.

The heart athlete: Artaud's affective athleticism

Doubles of the Artaudian body haunt a variety of performance practices of the twentieth century, and this next section now investigates Artaud's notion of the double in relation to the dance and theatre works discussed in this book. More specifically, we will closely examine the meaning and definition of the Artaudian double in relation to emotional memory and so-called "affective thought" (2005, p. 93). Let us begin with an extract from *The Theatre and Its Double*, in which Artaud writes on time and memory as they arise from the midst of our beating heart:

> Theatre has an effect on this Double, this ghostly effigy it moulds, and like all ghosts this apparition has a long memory. The heart's

> memory endures and an actor certainly thinks with his heart, for his heart holds sway [...] To understand the mystery of passionate time, a kind of musical tempo conducting its harmonic beat, is an aspect of the drama modern psychological theatre has certainly disregarded for some time. (2005, pp. 89–90)

Here, Artaud's concern for the performer as a "heart athlete" relates to an experience of time measured by the beating heart inside our chests. The pulse we feel is thus the barometer according to which we move and become alive as we breathe in and out in rhythmic patterns. As we have seen in Chapter 1, human life and consciousness emerge from this basic contraction and release of breath into our lungs. Birth is thus the first pathos we respond to as we begin to sense the world. When I say pathos, then I refer back to the concept introduced by the phenomenology of Michel Henry in Chapter 1; however, pathos also compares to Aristotle's theory of tragedy first outlined in the *Poetics* (335 BCE) and possibly an inspiration to later philosophers of phenomenology who were often well versed in the ancient texts. For Aristotle and the Greeks, pathos referred to the suffering of the tragic hero and involved a form of ritualistic cleansing and recognition which today we may think of as an early form of group therapy experienced by audiences in the theatre at the time.

It appears that Greek theatre had already picked up on the fact which neuroscientists like Damasio today describe as the "theatre of our mind" whereby we each imagine and enact our own little dramas of self, while at the same time interacting with the dramas of other people and media in front of us. While Greek tragedy emphasized the importance of myths as the foundation of Greek society and the Athenian city state to affirm the male audiences in their status of citizenship, suffering helped to maintain a status quo of law and awe (see Wiles, 2000). Pathos is therefore tied to the recognition of human humility in face of the Gods and fate, which according to the Greek myths was often predetermined and not for the Greek hero to interfere with or else he would be in trouble most often resulting in death or blindness as is the case in *King Oedipus* (Sophocles, 429 BC).

Bernard Waldenfels's phenomenology, however, refers to pathos in a much broader sense; it speaks of the fact that as humans we suffer from events such as birth and death in a rather indirect way beyond the control of our rational will (2011). There is not much willing in living, come to think of it, as we have only very little control over our primal bodily functions such as breathing, heartbeat and blood pressure, those that keep us healthy and alive – despite our efforts with diet control and regular exercise regimes. Waldenfels's point is that we are therefore much more passive in the way we respond to our situation as human beings on this planet than the legacy of Western rationalism would have us think.

Modernity, since the early enlightenment of the seventeenth and eighteenth centuries, promoted humans as active agents in control of their own fate supported by their command of language, rationalism and modern science. However, as the human mind became increasingly focused on thought as expressed in written words, politics also evolved in and around the lives of important men and – if unfortunately not always duly recognized – also women of course. And yet, as our lifetime is measured in heartbeats, there is an end to the subjective experience of our life as we know it autobiographically, no matter how great an individual's achievement over a lifespan may have been. While Western Christianity assumes that life comes to an end in death and that we will be judged on the grounds of our good deeds and sins, Eastern philosophies propose that there is a karmic debt we leave behind as a form of cosmically charged energy and that there are continuations of lives yet to be lived. However that may be, it appears that pathos is important as it shapes human experience and understanding of the world across an individual's lifetime.

When Artaud thus speaks of the "heart's memory", I suggest that he points towards the fact that our heart is the ticking clock inside our chest determining our life's beginning and end on very much its own accord. One way that we may hence define the complex concept of time is via this human experience of a lifetime measured by heartbeats as opposed to an eternal cosmic life force that beats on even as we ourselves no longer have a conscious memory and experience of our life after death. While most Western thought since the eighteenth-century enlightenment assumed that our memories end with our death, Artaud seems to suggest that the heart's memory goes beyond the individual life as its internal rhythms partake in a wider phenomenon of expending energy that can neither be produced on its own nor destroyed but only be transformed (see Noether, 1918). If the heart energy is thus our measure of time and a life lived, yet not fully consumed by it, then this opens a perspective according to which human experience is but a shadow, hence "double", to this ongoing cosmic life force.

Furthermore, if we recall Damasio's point that consciousness is but the mere "theatre of our emotions", then the roles we play are also impacted upon or affected by our emotional response to life. Maybe because we feel life most intimately bound up with the beating heart in our chest, many people will also locate the seat of their emotions in the heart which culturally becomes a symbol of love, compassion and affection. Also, as dancers, we move to the internal rhythms of our blood stream and breathing as we relate to the emotional depths of our felt reality. And yet, the moving itself is the initial precondition for us to feel and express emotion at all.

The Artaudian "double" hence becomes an aesthetic projection of self that reverberates with Sondra Fraleigh's phenomenological perspective on dance as "pure consciousness" and embodied response to feeling. As Fraleigh defines,

> This is a way of explaining that dance is most basically an aesthetic affirmation of the body and of life. The aesthetic underlies life as well as art, since it is itself founded in feeling as this extends into aisthesis, or sense perception. The lived body is a body of feeling, an interrelated system of life; and when it lives toward the world, it seeks an expressive body aesthetic, it manifests and does not withhold its life. Underlying its aesthetic surface, dance is an aesthetic projection of life. This phenomenal significance can be pointed out in the constancy of the lived ground of dance. (1987, p. 56)

In line with Artaud's theories, Fraleigh thus explains how life experience is shaped by feeling as it extends into sense perception and aesthetic projections of movement. A different way to account for the phenomenon of Artaudian "doubling" in performance derives from her phenomenological perspective on dance which considers feeling as a movement–response to being affected by the outside material world.

Henri Bergson on time: Memory and body image

Philosophers such as Henri Bergson (1859–1941) and Gilles Deleuze (1925–1995) were concerned to define our felt relationship to time as "duration" by which our past memory is prolonged into the present and evokes an intuited awareness of primordial existence in our bodies

(Bergson, 2005, pp. 243–244). The Artaudian "mystery of passionate time" hence creates meaning between matter and memory, if we follow Bergson's philosophical speculation. According to Bergson, matter refers to anything we perceive as outside our own body and even the body itself as we perceive it externally via the mirror image. However, our awareness of outside matter is intricately bound up with our immaterial inwardly felt response to it, and therefore Bergson suggests that memory plays a crucial part of how we recall images and matter from an inside/outside perspective. Henri Bergson provides us with an interesting perspective on the occurrence of inner psychological images as he conceives of matter as "an existence placed halfway between the 'thing' and the 'representation'" (2005, p. 10) and therefore grasped "in the form of images" (2005, p. 26).

The body is thus one such memory-image, however central to our current perception of matter around us. While perception generally takes place in the present, it involves, according to Bergson, "a certain duration [...] an effort of memory which prolongs, one into another, a plurality of moments" (2005, p. 34) whereby our memory of the past encapsulated by the soul continuously impacts on our perception of our body in the present. He explains,

> Every perception fills a certain depth of duration, prolongs the past into the present, and thereby partakes of memory. So that if we take perception, in its concrete form, as a synthesis of pure memory and pure perception, that is to say, of mind and matter, we compress within its narrowest limits the problem of the union of soul and body. (2005, pp. 243–244)

For Bergson our awareness of the past is thus recollected via the capacity of our mind – which he calls "spirit" – to recall outside matter ("the world") as an inside image connected to our soul. For example, once we see a tree, the concept of tree stays with us as an inner image even if the actual tree is no longer there. It seems that Bergson preferred the word "spirit" rather than "mind", because it implies a somewhat religious overtone of sacred mystery and awe towards consciousness as our lived capacity for feeling-toned perception in the first place which as such predates and outlives our actual birth as humans.

For Bergson, to realize that the human mind can actually synthesize different temporalities in the instant of a moment thereby evoking memories from the past and also projecting them forward to form our future responses does indeed imply that human core-consciousness, somatically located in our spine which interconnects the autonomous nervous system (ANS) with the brain, transcends our own limited understanding of it. But not only does the body's response synthesize the perception as such, it is also informed by a felt response which Bergson's thinking resolves in the ultimate union of body and soul. While the body makes up for the perceptual apparatus being the vessel of mind, organs, blood, etc., the soul marks our felt subjectivity evoked by it. As an "instrument of action" (Bergson, 2005, p. 225), the body thus projects images of our past and those contained by the concept of soul into the future by continuously extending corporeal memory into present consciousness (Bergson, 2005, pp. 78–79).

For Bergson inner psychological images are thus placed as an intermediary between a thing ("matter") of the outside world and its representation ("memory"). He thus argues against idealist/realist distinctions between existence and appearance by turning his attention to matter itself before that separation (Bergson, 2005, pp. 9–10). Bergson is therefore an important precursor of phenomenology but also neuroscience as he was interested in the relationship of matter and consciousness, the functions of our medullary system (spinal cord) and the brain for recollection and memory (Bergson, 2005, pp. 28–29). According to Bergson, perception is an effort of memory (Bergson, 2005, p. 34) that coincides with the body (Bergson, 2005, p. 74) and its motor habits (Bergson, 2005, p. 225). He explains,

> The body retains motor habits capable of acting the past over again; it can resume attitudes in which the past will insert itself; or, again, by the repetition of certain cerebral phenomena, which have prolonged former perceptions, it can furnish to remembrance a point of attachment with the actual, a means of recovering its lost influence upon present reality [...] (2005, pp. 225–226)

Perception is thus performing a choice by eliminating "from the totality of images" those that make up our body (Bergson, 2005, pp. 228–229). We perceive in actions, and whereas the past is experienced as an idea, Bergson calls the present "ideo-motor" (2005, pp. 68–69). He elaborates on how this perspective collapses our distinction between recollection and perception (2005, pp. 68–69). As a consequence, personal existence is "intimately bound up" with affection and the soul as they gradually transform feeling into representation and concept both founded on subjective experience (Bergson, 2005, pp. 53–54). And yet the line between affection and its perception as representation is thin as again they meet on the surface of the body:

> Between the affection felt and the image perceived there is this difference, that the affection is within our body, the image outside our body. And that is why the surface of our body, the common limit of this and of other bodies, is given to us in the form both of sensation and of an image. (Bergson, 2005, p. 234)

Hence, Bergson conceives of memory as, in principle, "absolutely independent of matter" and, therefore, irrevocably bound up with spirit as an independent reality (2005, pp. 73–74). And yet there is reciprocity of action between the two at the point of duration which is the instance of time each perception will take by prolonging "the past into the present, and thereby partak[ing] of memory" (Bergson, 2005, pp. 243–244). In that sense, perception synthesizes pure memory, and pure perception of mind and matter aligns it with the problem of the union of body and soul (Bergson, 2005, pp. 243–244).

However, it appears doubtful whether anything about the existence of pure memory or the soul can be ascertained beyond its value as an axiomatic principle or felt truth. As Bergson points out, our perception of the present is in fact "one foot in my past and another in my future" if we look at it from the point of duration (2005, pp. 137–138). The present is also per definition "sensori-motor" which means that it is "both sensation and movement" prolonged in action (Bergson, 2005, p. 138). Being present thus "consists in the consciousness I have of my body" and "appears to me a thing absolutely determined, and contrasting with my past" (Bergson, 2005, p. 138). This is further complicated by the dictum that "*[p]ractically, we perceive only the past*, the pure present being the invisible progress of the past gnawing into the future" (Bergson, 2005, p. 150). For Bergson Western body–mind dualism is therefore primarily a problem of how we define time. He explains,

> [W]e can understand that spirit can rest upon matter and, consequently, unite with it in the act of pure perception, yet nevertheless be radically distinct from it. It is distinct from matter in that it is,

> even then, memory, that is to say, a synthesis of past and present with a view to the future, in that it contracts the moments of this matter in order to use them to manifest itself by actions which are the final aim of its union with the body. We were right, then, when we said, at the beginning of this book, that the distinction between body and mind must be established in terms not of space but of time. (Bergson, 2005, p. 220)

To summarize Henri Bergson's thought on time and memory and bring it back to Artaud's concept of the heart athlete and passionate time, it is important for us to realize that both Artaud and Bergson conceive of the body as our central image-making vehicle which allows us to make sense of ourselves and the world by fully connecting the inside-out relatedness of our conscious experience.

Hence Artaud's suggestion that theatre make a claim on the corporeal memory of "passionate time" is invested in movement precisely because it materializes the spiritual dimension of affective thought and memory in the durational presence of embodied time. Whether in response to images of nature, collective myth or story-telling, affective sensation constitutes the "source of movement" located in the "body, [which] constitutes at every moment, [...] a section of the universal becoming" (Bergson, 2005, pp. 151–152). Affective athleticism as an experience of affective intensity is thus a sensation stored within the body and articulated in movement, oftentimes referred to as intuition or instinct. At the intersection of spirit and matter, the Artaudian "heart athlete" thus presents a "double" per definition as she simultaneously enacts the present matter of our past recollections of feeling. In that sense, a theatre of cruelty will thus always converse with history and its doubles in dance and performance.

1947/48: *To Have Done with the Judgement of God* or Artaud's last dance

In 1947 Fernand Pouey, head of dramatic and literary broadcasts for French National Radio, commissioned Artaud to work on a radio play which became *To Have Done with the Judgement of God*. This was recorded between 22 and 29 November 1947 and on 16 January 1948 (Barber, 1993, pp. 150–152). As Rick Dolphijn suggests, we may look at this text as a comment "on the state of the (Western) world" (2011, p. 19), even more so as it was finished three years after the end of the Second World War and about a year before the Universal Declaration of Human Rights on 10 December 1948. In 2015, Artaud's radio play reads like an uncanny premonition of historical events oddly fulfilled. Lucidly, he attacks American capitalism and prophesizes future wars being fought over natural resources to maintain high consumerist culture through and beyond the Cold War conflict with Russia as quoted here:

> For war is wonderful, isn't it?/ For it's war, isn't it, that the Americans have been preparing for/ and are preparing for this way step by step./ In order to defend this senseless manufacture from all competition that could not fail to arise on all sides,/ one must have soldiers, armies, airplanes, battleships,/ hence this sperm/ which it seems the governments of America have had the ef-/ frontery to think of./ For we have more than one enemy/ lying in wait for us, my son,/ we, the born capitalists [...]. (1976, p. 556).

Artaud's *To Have Done With the Judgement of God* points towards the increasing objectification of the body in late capitalist culture which he aligns with the rule of representation that condemned his surrealist writing style and banished the actual broadcasting of the radio play just a day before it was supposed to go on air on 2 February 1948 (Barber, 1993, p. 157). At the same time *To Have Done With the Judgement of God* writes dance into theatre as the recording envisions a "body-without-organs" (BwO) announcing the spiritual–energetic intensity of the counter-cultural street protests yet to come, when in 1968 performance art and dance took over street politics (see Barber, 2013).

Based on Artaud's perspective on non-Western rituals as he had witnessed among the Tarahumaras and his travels to Mexico, the section titled "the dance of Tutuguri" describes a communal circle dance to do away with "the judgement of God" and its colonialist politics of the cross. Performed by six men and a seventh symbolizing the sun, the described dance venerates the earth accompanied by "the anguish of a drum and a long trumpet" while the performers are "lying down,/ rolling level with the ground,/" to then "leap up one by one like sunflowers,/ not like suns/ but turning earths/ water lilies,/ and each leap/ corresponds to the increasingly somber/ and restrained/ gong of the drum [...]" (1976, p. 558). The dance outlined here appears as a poetic ritual at the end of which a "body without organs" emerges to free consciousness from the limitations of the human body. Artaud envisions ritualistic trance as a lived experience of liminality between life and death to abolish the notion of death as it exists in the Christian model of resurrection. He thereby asserts the presence of death in life to re-establish a spiritual continuum between the living and the dead prevalent in many premodern cultural cosmologies. To abolish the cross then suggests that an Artaudian performance – just like the dance of the Tutuguri – does not try to "conquer" but resurrect those unconscious liminal powers essential to earthly life. As Dolphijn further explains,

> Artaud states that cleaning the body of its incorporated Christianity requires that we break through the Christian Trinity in search of the unknown of the body/the unconscious of thought. The BwO. Only in this way can we find our organic culture. (2011, p. 30)

The dance of the Tutuguri, like all dance, thus brings forth the "unconscious of thought" or to recall Fraleigh's point from Chapter 1 "founds the meaning that words name" (1987, p. 73). In that sense dance allows for "autorepresentation" as Derrida suggests for Artaud's theatre, when he writes,

> [...] Artaud insists upon the productive images without which there would be no theatre (theaomai) – but whose visibility does not consist of a spectacle mounted by the discourse of the master. Representation, then, as the autopresentation of pure visibility and even pure sensibility. (Derrida, 1997 [1978], p. 238)

Artaud's writing of dance into theatre is thus based on the felt core-conscious body-response which is, as a matter of fact ,coincidental with Bergson's notion of the spirit/soul to exist beyond our lived autobiographical self. The BwO then is precisely consciousness as it opens up towards infinity. As Artaud poses the question in the section titled "The Question Arises ...":

> What makes it serious/ is that we know/ that after the order/ of this world/ there is another./ What is it like?/ We do not know./ The number and order of possible suppositions in/ this realm/ is precisely/ infinity!/ And what is infinity?/ That is precisely what we do not know!/ It is a word/ that we use/ to indicate/ the opening/ of our

> consciousness/ toward possibility/ beyond measure,/ tireless and beyond measure. (1976, pp. 562–563)

In this passage Artaud claims that the infinite realm of thought is first experienced as a form of intuited knowledge – or in Damasio's terms emotional response – that is subsequently expressed in sounds, movement, drawing and language. To open one's consciousness to a "possibility beyond measure" draws from the same intuitive impulse we call freedom in dance because it transcends the notion of the everyday self and its representations. The dancer's expressive quality is beyond the merely human as he or she taps into the creative source of her core self and its cosmic movement potential.

Artaud must have realized the force of such performance as he had first recognized it in the transcendental power of Balinese dance theatre as well as among the Tarahumara people. The Balinese classical temple dance and the other indigenous dance rituals oddly matched Artaud's own spells of drug-induced hallucination and clarity whereby a layer of consciousness situated beyond life and death made itself visible. Later, the electroshock treatment at Rodez brought the out-of-body experience even closer whereby Artaud's mind expanded beyond the limitations of the deceasing body carcass. Artaud's later drawings and writings speak to this experience of mind expansion as the artist's ultimate resort to freedom in a society of psychiatric incarceration. The two world wars had brought out the worst in humankind: there was disrespect of the sacredness of life and the planet that resulted in mass murders and the death machine of the Nazi concentration camps. "God", in the Western world, was no longer worshipped as the sacred source of life inside each human being, but was represented as a travesty of fascistic power and dictatorship closely aligned with the colonialist–capitalist project of global expansion and the war over resources.

Modernity and Western capitalism in particular had thus severed the ancestral connection to life's energy disrespected under the perverted rational judgement of a personified dictator–God representative of a paternalistic ideology of colonialist power and oppression. Artaud's raving battle cry derived from a place of heartfelt pain and suffering questioning the hubris at the core of post-Enlightenment Western civilization and rationalism. The schizophrenia and depression opened a place for him to look beyond and deeper inside the workings of the human mind, and his writings read like the broken mirror image that Lacan's psychology brought to the fore at the time (see Barber, 2013). If the history of Western individualism and consumer society should prove to hold ever more tightly to the figure represented by the mirror, Artaud's writings and drawings tell us otherwise. Here we are drawn inside ourselves where our own subjective truth of pain and joy resides. If we dance for ourselves – improvising – the same energy becomes manifest as it spills outward into movement. Hence, the liberation that Artaud's *To Have Done with the Judgement of God* calls for is to shift focus away from the mirror image that the theatre and society of his time so ardently defended so as to start dancing the "wrong side out" finding and expressing our own truths and creative potential. As the ending of Artaud's radio play reveals,

> For you can tie me up if you wish,/ but there is nothing more useless than an organ./ When you will have made him a body without organs,/ then you will have delivered him from all his automatic reactions/ and restored him to his true freedom./ Then you will teach him again to dance wrong side out/ as in the frenzy of dance halls/ and this wrong side out will be his real place. (1976, p. 571)

In the following chapters we will see examples of what "dancing the wrong side out" may be as we move along several examples of twentieth-century theatre and dance performances, but before we do, let us turn to another forefather of twentieth-century dance theatre: Bertolt Brecht.

Study Questions:

1. How does Artaud's suffering from schizophrenia impact on his theory of theatre?
2. What was the impact of Balinese dance theatre for Artaud – are there commonalities between his "theatre of cruelty" and dance?
3. To what extent does spirituality inform his concept of theatre? Is that the same for dance?
4. What constitutes Artaud's idea of the performer as "heart athlete"? Does it relate to dance and emotion as defined in the previous chapter?
5. How can Henri Bergson's reflection on time and duration help us understand the notion of Artaud's "double"?
6. What is the relationship between body image and memory?

3 Choreographing Gestus

Bertolt Brecht and the Evolution of Epic Theatre

The origins of epic theatre: Erwin Piscator (1893–1966)

Erwin Friedrich Max Piscator was born on 17 December 1893 at the village of Ulm near Wetzlar. He was son to Carl Piscator, a merchant, and Antonia Laperose. The family moved to Marburg, where he attended school until 1913 before he went to Munich where he took up his early studies in German, philosophy and art history. In August 1914 the First World War started and its gruesome brutality affected a whole generation of young soldiers who would never recover if they were lucky enough to survive it. For the young Erwin Piscator the experience as a soldier in the First World War became decisive for his future commitment to political theatre. As he recalls this memory in *The Political Theatre* (published in German as *Das Politische Theater* 1929) and as we may learn from his diaries kept during the war, this experience changed his outlook on his profession as an actor forever after:

> The moment I uttered the word actor among the exploding shells, the whole profession for which I had struggled so hard and which I held so dear in common with all art, seemed so comical, so stupid, so ridiculous, so grotesquely false, in short so ill-suited to the situation, so irrelevant to my life, to our life, to life in this day and age, that I was less afraid of the flying shells than I was ashamed of my profession. (1980, pp. 13–14)

Between 1914 and 1918 Piscator conducted productions for the army theatre units and published several anti-war poems in the critical Berlin magazine *Die Aktion* during the years 1915 and 1916. Piscator marks the beginning of a generation of theatre makers influenced by the traumatic experience of the Great War and hence committed to art that subscribed to a pacifist ethics of societal change. Thousands had been gassed in the trenches, and the horror spurred Piscator's future prospects for a revolutionary theatre to fight the cause of the common man to understand the political circumstances of the time.

During the turbulent years and political upheavals of the Weimar Republic, Piscator joined the Tribunal theatre (Das Tribunal) in Königsberg 1919/20 following the November Revolution and the murders of Rosa Luxemburg and Karl Liebknecht, the two leading politicians of the Communist Party (KPD). Piscator, an ardent communist, became a member of the Spartacus group, which was one of the splinter groups of the divided left wing at that time. Here, Piscator's amateur group staged mostly progressive plays from the expressionist repertoire (Wedekind, Kaiser, Strindberg) and somewhat failed his Marxist-oriented politics as his audiences were mostly bourgeois and did not draw from the proletarian masses.

As a consequence, Piscator moved to Berlin where in September 1920 he founded his Proletarian Theatre (Proletarisches Theater). Audiences were addressed as "Comrades!" and most performances were held for working-class spectators in beer halls and meeting rooms. Rather than producing established plays from the expressionist repertoire, the group performed improvised scripts and party propaganda to have an immediate political impact. Proletarian theatre of the time served as a direct political tool close to the Russian Agitprop model, a means to communicate and uplift the working-class masses rather than to feed a bourgeois notion of entertainment (see Innes, 1972, pp. 20–22).

Agitprop theatre feeds on the very basic elements of theatre based in the ancient art of communal storytelling, where a central speaker is surrounded by an encircling audience. This could be a simple market place or a more elaborate edifice, like the town meeting hall, but essentially the basic emotive eye-to-eye communication remains the same, and Agitprop was effectively used by the Russian Communists after the Revolution to spread news to the peasant masses in the rural areas of the vast country. Playing without costumes, curtains or scenery, the Agitprop performances used speech, song, dance and gymnastics to dramatize texts that were taken from actual news items and proved to be a successful means of party propaganda.

Piscator's Proletarian Theatre may therefore be seen as a forerunner to Agitprop and was sponsored by the German Communist Party as Piscator's political theatre of the 1920s broke ground for the spread of Communist party politics in Germany. Performances were held in beer and festival halls where the stage was at best a low platform; the whole illusionist scenery of the professional theatre was naturally lacking and most often actors did not have a choice but to enter the stage from the midst of the audience. While Piscator returned in a sense to the very basic elements of the medieval platform stages, he also claimed that he discovered the basic principles of epic theatre by accident or rather through practical exploration and improvisation. As Maria Ley-Piscator recalls in her memoir *The Piscator Experiment*:

> Epic Theatre, too, was born out of necessity. It happened. It was not invented in the quiet study of a playwright polishing theatrical history. It was born in the street ... in the turmoil of a city impoverished by war and inflation, and in the life of a roving theatrical company, performing in halls and meeting places in the suburbs ... (1967, pp. 11–12)

Compared to Bertolt Brecht as the poet–theoretician, Erwin Piscator is often referred to as the engineer of the epic theatre as he emphasized the scenic elements of the staging. In both concepts of epic theatre though – and after all Bertolt Brecht started his early career with the Piscatorbühne and has credited Piscator's influence on his own development of epic theatre and alienation effects – the idea of the play involves far more than the plot line itself, in the sense that the overall scenic composition needs to reveal the whole complex relation of the human being to the world.

Epic theatre I: Scenic composition and movement image

Epic theatre starts from the premise of scenic composition, whereby the actors create a physical relationship that embodies the politics of the character constellation. It is such dramatic and visual economy that defines epic theatre rather than the dramatic text to the effect that each theatrical element serves as a metonym of the larger political conflict.

In that sense then, epic theatre "reflects a mode of thinking, acting, perceiving and living of a [particular historical] period [and class constellation]" (Ley-Piscator, 1967, pp. 14–15). While the traumatic experience of the Great War and the ongoing working-class street fights during the Weimar Republic were also important influences on Piscator's theatrical development of epic theatre in terms of its political message, the impact of modernization, industrialization and technology were just as important in terms of their aesthetic exploration of form in the overall shaping of his artistic vision of a political theatre of the future.

As the so-called father of "analytical-technical scenery", Piscator became the director of a collective theatrical collaboration of engaged artists, joined by Bertolt Brecht (poet), George Grosz (satiric painter of the "New Sobriety"), Ernst Toller (socialist playwright) and Walter Gropius (leading architect of the Bauhaus' "art and technology – a new unity" slogan) to name but the most renowned. Together they achieved an experimental form of avant-garde theatre to introduce a complex blend of technology and drama as climaxed in Piscator's best remembered productions of Ernst Toller's *Hoppla, We Live* and *The Good Soldier Schwejk*, starring the famous Austrian actor Max Pallenberg.

The opening of Toller's *Hoppla, We Live* at the Theater am Nollendorfplatz – from then on also to be known as "Piscatorbühne" because of the independent company he now worked with – marked a turning point in Piscator's career. The play, which is difficult to trace, since we have no documented script available any longer, apparently is the story of a man who is convicted of political crime and spends ten years in a lunatic asylum from where he is released at the beginning of the play. As the play develops, he cannot make sense of the world around him any longer, and he finds the world itself increasingly insane. Confronted by the political upheavals of the Weimar Republic during the 1920s, the protagonist is yet again imprisoned. Desperate to escape insanity, he tragically hangs himself in the end.

The production, however, was noticed less for its expressionistic take on the entrapped individual in modern society than for Piscator's stage technological inventions. Thus the ten years in prison were captured by a newsreel flashback projection of the Russian Revolution (1917), the Czar's violent death and the end of the First World War (1918), the Versailles Treaty (1919), Mussolini's march on Rome (1922) and Hitler's beer hall putsch at Munich (1923) and imprisonment, where he wrote his infamous *Mein Kampf*. Traugott Müller's four-tiered stage structure was individually lit for each scene in the various ministerial offices and the hotel rooms, whereas larger episodes were played across the whole stage, with film excerpts and illustrations projected. There was singing during the second half of the play as well as live piano and other surprising sound effects; text projections were also introduced to an astounding and politically controversial effect as some of the conservative critics of the time observed.

Simultaneous staging and montage expressed Piscator's increasing dissatisfaction with the prevalent naturalism of the time and reflected on new perceptions of time and space as made possible by the new media: radio and film. Together with his fellow collaborators at the Piscatorbühne he sought to surpass naturalism's limitations through a heightened critical sense of realism in combining theatrical and filmic conventions of the moving image. Epic theatre thus mobilizes the spectator's gaze as it heightens our overall perception of events. Piscator's goal was to achieve a "moving path" in terms of a dynamic interaction between the observer and the observed, as he saw it at work also in the mural paintings of Orozco and the early films of Sergei Eisenstein (1898–1948):

> It's like a montage film, a magnificent, colorful film. Montage of action, of thought, of conflict – a montage of drama. It is a blending of things, people and events. What a succession of images, to illustrate the association of ideas, clear as headlines! What a release from petrified painting! It is not accidental that the spiritual metamorphosis in the arts comes at the same time as the technical transformation of its tools. It is the same in the theatre. (Ley-Piscator, 1967, pp. 54–55)

Whereas nineteenth-century naturalism and realism sought to render a face-value copy of photographic reality, epic theatre emphasized theatrical construction in its proclaimed search for dialectical truth. The technique was thus based on demonstration rather than fictional sentimentality, and the focus on the event itself became more important than the plot. The demonstration of the facts of life became the emphasis rather than the revelation of psychological mysteries. "Historic drama, to interest us today", so Piscator argued, "cannot be the tragedy of some hero, but must be the political document of the age" (Ley-Piscator, 1967, p. 84).

In a sense, the film and documentary material visually assumed the importance of the antique dancing chorus in these epic plays, as it commented on the dramatic action and idealistic sequences portrayed. Together with Gropius Piscator outlined plans for a concept of "total theatre", that is, a continued architectural blend of film and drama in theatre design to integrate simultaneous staging and montage technique as a direct spatial response to the changed patterns of modernization, as it redefined and to some extent dissolved the classical Aristotelian unity of former notions of dramatic treatment of time and space. Piscator explained his early search as such:

> We apply to art the idea of relativity. We have abstract art in painting. We have a twelve-tone scale in music. But whatever one thinks of these new forms, they are scarcely employed in the theatre of today. (Ley-Piscator, 1967, p. 17)

Though, the theatre itself has never been realized and Piscator, for his productions at the Theater am Nollendorfplatz, had to make do with the existing feudalistic structures of the court theatre's proscenium stage which was clearly limiting and obviously lacking his and Gropius's experimental vision. As Gropius summarizes the function of such scenic revision and design:

> The aim of this theater is no longer to accumulate a collection of fanciful technical apparatus and gimmickry; everything is a means to an end: the end is to draw the spectator into the middle of the scenic events, to make him part of the space in which the events are taking place and prevent him from escaping from them under cover of the curtain. In addition, a theater architect is bound in my opinion by a duty to make the stage instrument as impersonal, responsive and versatile as possible, so that the various directors are free to develop their various artistic concepts. (Piscator, 1980, p. 183)

Piscator's experiments as well as Gropius's architectural designs are evidence that the theatre managed to synthesize and critically comment on the perceptive changes evoked by the new media technologies. Between the two world wars, reality was already far more complex than theatrical realism – whether on stage or in the cinema – would have its audiences believe. Instead of linear concepts of time and space, simultaneity and relativity were increasingly explored through the choreography of movement and image. In that sense, epic theatre's scenic composition aligns itself with movement choreography as the performers, projections, sound and improvisation had to be collaboratively designed and composed. As J. L. Styan comments on Piscator's political use of film in the theatre, it

> [...] can be timed to support, expand or comment on the stage action, the images on the stage and on the screens even suggesting cause and effect – the most commonplace arrangement was to have a political speech delivered on stage, while behind the speaker the screen showed, say, the resulting horrors of the battlefield. In this way, the film could make a quick, generalized, usually emotive, statement at a moment's notice, and was particularly useful in illustrating the rambling historical narratives Piscator chose, where the general image was made to balance the particularity of the lines. (1981, p. 131)

Consequently, Piscator's innovative use of technological apparatuses in the theatre presented itself as an aesthetic shock far beyond the mere introduction of new media technology: in the sense that total theatre provided its audiences with a meta comment on changed patterns of perception, news transmission and politics.

To summarize, epic theatre in Piscator's early definition disregarded the classical Aristotelian unities of time and place as much as the nineteenth-century realistic conventions of the proscenium stage or so-called five-act well-made play. Rather, epic theatre emphasized scenic composition to highlight its underlying political themes to allow the spectator to draw his or her own political conclusions from the historical facts and events presented on stage. Although performers acted rather than danced in these productions, they were carefully choreographed as part of the overall scenic image. Movements also often derived from improvisation – not unlike those discovered by modern dance at the time – and were in direct dialogue with the overall political message sought to be conveyed. Piscator's use of machinery furthermore reflected the technological innovations of modern scientific society (screens, news materials and films), and simultaneous projection served as a narrative device to comment upon the complexity of modern life as reality was increasingly perceived through the filter of the emerging propaganda machinery of mass media. Newsreels and still photographs, as well as Grosz's satiric cartoons provided critical commentary and helped the actor to assume an anti-naturalistic distance in creating the desired objectivity as the narrator of his or her part. Increasingly, this method made use of everyday objects and props to evoke "gestus", the critical term Brecht then introduced to define a politics of embodiment underlying his dramatic oeuvre.

Epic theatre II: Choreographing gestus – The legacy of Bertolt Brecht (1898–1956)

Bertolt Brecht's indebtedness to Piscator becomes evident in his use of storytelling, commentary, title projections and song to support the mechanical stage apparatus of his theatre, though he came to focus on the parable play and its moral dilemma to highlight his dramatic writing as well as his elaboration of the particular role of the actor in his theatre. Key aspects of Brecht's theory and practice of theatre were based on the notion of epic theatre, a term that he replaced with dialectical theatre later on in his career, as he surpassed Piscator's original conceptualization of the term. Brecht's continued theatrical explorations thus redefined Piscator's earlier theory of epic performance over the years. For Brecht the actor's gestus was more important than the latest stage technology and stayed at the heart of his political project. It is therefore no coincidence, when Brecht pleads for a theatre with more choreography in his "Short Organon for Theatre": "Anyhow, a theatre where everything depends on the gest cannot do without choreography. Elegant movement and graceful grouping, for a start, can alienate, and inventive miming greatly helps the story" (Willet, 1964, p. 204).

In Brecht's early writings, the epic theatre is characterized as the non-Aristotelian theatre, not only in terms of its disregard of the unity of time and place, but more importantly as it was against the bourgeois-ideological appropriation of the tragic form in its illusionist realism. Aristotelian drama in Brecht's reading is representative of tragedy, because it depicts the tragic hero or heroine as facing next to insurmountable obstacles determined by their social or mytho-religious fate. It is therefore an expression of reactionary bourgeois morality, Brecht argues, because the tragic plot is irrevocably linked to the politics of the status quo. Consequently, Brecht's epic drama addressed the changing dynamics of social order in the early years of the Weimar Republic, whereas tragedy and the realist well-made play adhered to conservative monarchical structures. However, epic theatre was not per se against emotion. Rather, Brecht's epic theatre sought to do away with the conventional way in which emotions were used in realism to manipulate audience response, when spectators were simply swept away by identifying with the character's actions.

By contrast, emotions in epic theatre are therefore rather more examined than shared with the audience in the sense that the spectator is always positioned at a distance. The spectators do not feel as if they are in the role of the character but rather assume, for example, the part of the detective who tries to analyse the characters' situation by asking questions about their actions and circumstances. Important for Brecht's Marxist concept is the working of dialectics in his theatre to overcome the sociopolitical contradiction and injustice. The actor's role is paramount in achieving this effect and appears far more important than is often acknowledged. As Brecht first put it in his canonical essay "The Street Scene: A Basic Model for an Epic Theatre",

> [T]he theatre only has to develop a technique for submitting emotions to the spectator's criticism. Of course this does not mean that the spectator must be barred on principle from sharing certain emotions that are put before him; none the less to communicate emotions is only one particular form (phase, consequence) for criticism. The theatre's demonstrator, the actor, must apply a technique which will let him reproduce the tone of the subject demonstrated with a certain reserve, with detachment (so that the spectator can say: "He's getting excited – in vain, too late, at last ..."etc.). In short, the actor must remain a demonstrator; he must present the person demonstrated as a stranger, he must suppress the "he did that, he said that" element in his performance. He must not go so far as to be wholly transformed into the person demonstrated. (Willett, 1964, p. 125)

Demonstration in the sense of a scientific experiment is thus the key to Brecht's theatre and acting theory. The notion of "gestus" in the combined sense of "gist and actions" (Willett, 1964) implies the sociological dimension of certain gestures not unlike the notion of "habitus" defined by sociologist Pierre Bourdieu (1930–2002) in his *Outline of a Theory of Practice* (1977, pp. 72–95). As Ana Sanchez-Colberg has argued,

> In Brechtian theatre the "body politic" is encapsulated within the A-Effekt, the process of theatrical presentation by which the formation of the theatrical "gestus" aims to discover "social relationships" which gave rise to it and, thus, reveal its social construction. [...] With Brecht one encounters a first attempt at a revolution of language both verbal and theatrical which will lead (in later generations) to a revolution of that language as it is embodied. Epic theatre techniques are geared to re-emphasize (and, therefore, defamiliarize) the process of language construction. (1996, p. 41)

"Gestus" consequently refers to a characteristic posture and attitude of a character as it relates to his social position in society. Alienation or "Verfremdung" as the main device of epic theatre ultimately results from the dialectical separation of elements in a non-linear, narrative demonstration of the plot. The repertoire of alienation devices, acting, singing, projections, chorus, etc., serves the production of double perspective: to point to the action's contradictions and to show the audiences alternative perceptions of history.

Helene Weigel as Mother Courage, Deutsches Theater Berlin, 1949

Helene Weigel's lead as Mother Courage in the 1949 production, which established the Berlin Ensemble at the Deutsches Theater Berlin, is legendary. For years to follow, it became the company's repertory production and played over four hundred times; it was awarded, filmed and photographed; and stamps appeared in its honour with Weigel's countenance, and the wagon became the most renowned theatre prop of all time (Kupke, 1981, p. 9). In 1949 theatre audiences in Berlin would have had a real sense of the aftermath of the war, as the Berliner Ensemble performed among the debris and devastation of bombed houses, death and destruction all around (Kupke, 1977, p. 8). The pathos of war was a scenario each spectator had already internalized as an image and experience that was becoming part of the scenic action at that time and somewhat completed the intended dialectics of *Mother Courage* performed in 1949. The challenge for contemporary productions therefore consists in choreographing such gestic images to call upon embodied memory and experience for the spectator, yet avoiding a naturalistic aesthetic.

Brecht's "Modellbuch zur Auffuehrung 1949" serves as a notation score to highlight the way he was working with Helene Weigel on the character. Model books consisted of 450–600 still photographs accompanied by critical commentary and observation documented during the rehearsal process (Weigel, 1952, p. 294). The attempt was to capture entrances and exits, as well as selected movements and gestures that conveyed the plot and underlying gestus ("Grundgestus") of the play. "Gestus" thus consists of the interplay of characters and groups in their movement, composition of plot in smaller scenic actions, characterization of roles and meaning of events (Weigel, 1952, p. 296). Directing assistants took notes on the choreography (positions and groups), intonations, social criticism, comic and tragic moments, etc. (Weigel, 1952, p. 296). Brecht's style of directing was described as working from a "child's perspective [...] directing twigs toward the stream so that they can start to flow" to allow the actor's freedom to explore and find appropriate movement and gestic material (Weigel, 1952, p. 130).

Movement improvisation became a key element for the actors to find the right movement and gesture to convey the story in a truthful manner, and it is also known to what extent Weigel used realistic props to that effect (Weigel, 1952, p. 130). Such gestic truth is therefore not evidenced by the dramatic text but consists in the human interaction taking place between the actors on stage. Brecht's attention was on detail and scenic image: colours, movement arrangement and gestures so that in each performance something new could be discovered (Weigel, 1952, p. 131). The evidence provided by Brecht's *Modellbuch* – a notation the Berliner Ensemble also kept for other productions – indicates the extent to which his role as director assumed much of the function of a choreographer or film director to assure the proper alignment of movement and space.

In *Mother Courage* the scenic arrangement evolved from the circular rotation of the waggon across the empty stage which evoked the cyclic repetition of war over the centuries. The movement furthermore encapsulates the main idea the play presents for audience examination as outlined by Brecht: "That in wartime the big profits are not made by little people. That war, which is a continuation of business by other means, makes the human virtues fatal even to their possessors. That no sacrifice is too great for the struggle against war" (Hecht, 1982, p. 9 [my translation]). As a chronicle of the Thirty Years' War, *Mother Courage* presents history from the perspective of a working woman's struggle for profit and survival. Her life evolves from a series of business transactions that leaves her childless in the end as she loses her family – first her sons then her daughter – to the war. Unlike the model of classical tragedy, however, her human suffering is always portrayed as the outcome of a particular political situation rather than her personal fate. Thus, politics drives her towards war and business rather than her own personal greed, although that may also come into the equation. As Roland Barthes's photo essay on the 1949 production highlights,

> The objective meaning of the play is what Brecht calls the social gesture, and that is the political test; I want to show how the detail of the gesture has a political meaning, rendering properly and correctly the differing alienation of the roles. [...] This is what distancing is: to fulfill the true purpose of a play where the meaning is no longer the actor's truth, but the political relationship of situations. (1967, p. 45)

The choreographic constellation or scenic "arrangement" is therefore crucial to help create the gestic narrative structure via movement and stillness rather than suggestive emotional involvement or verbal diction. Brecht's *Modellbuch* indicates specified "walks and group arrangements", whereby actors move across the diagonals, centre and front of stage to demonstrate the gestic nature of the political constellation that influences their actions (Weigel, 1952, p. 234). Walks and gestures are crucial for the overall narration of the plot. In 1949 Helene Weigel's embodiment of the silent scream responded to the rifle shots in the distance as an expression of her inner pain and shame to have lost her son Schweizerkas. The audience could only see her wide open mouth but did not hear anything, she then turned around and froze into a backwards facing pose with her shoulders up, torso extended and gaze facing upward (Kupke, 1981, pp. 114–115).

Throughout Brecht's 1949 production of *Mother Courage,* Helene Weigel's choreographed "gestus" – as documented by the photographs – presents an expression of a heightened naturalism, which she derived from close examination of social reality in her choice of props and movement. However, whereas naturalism is highly illusionistic in its representational obsession to provide imagistic detail of the milieu as to disguise its constructedness, the Brechtian approach presents the natural as constructed, that is, precisely to be questioned in its deterministic status quo. The Brechtian stage is empty and consciously filled with

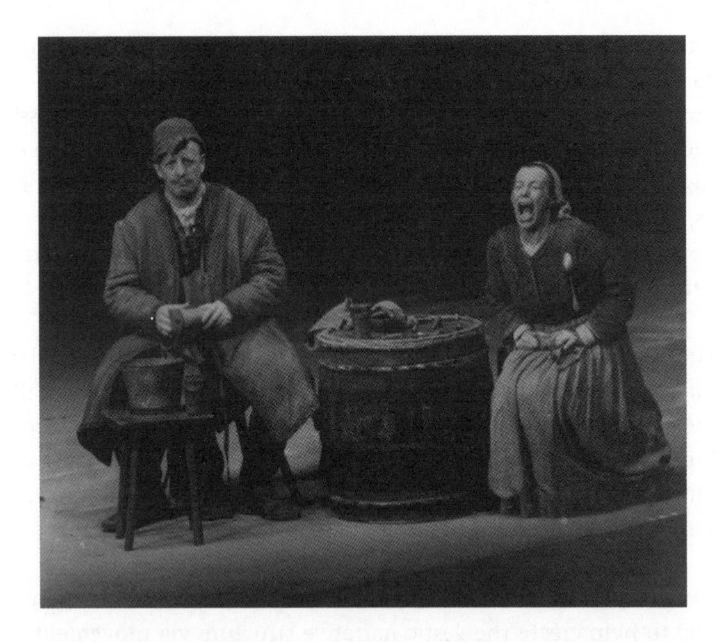

Helene Weigel as Mother Courage, © Akademie der Künste, Berlin, Bertolt-Brecht-Archiv FA 50/239, Photo: Hainer Hill

sparse props and other devices to always make this point. When Helene Weigel opens her mouth to a scream without sound, she gives an expressionistic image of pain that she possibly observed from a photograph of a woman who had lost her child, yet she heightens it by withholding the expected sound. Similarly, Therese Giehse's performance in Brecht's *The Mother* created gestus through her movements and actions that captured a common-sense wit of the working class.

Study Questions:

1. How does Piscator's scenic composition compare to choreography?
2. What is the importance of *gestus* for Brecht's theatre?
3. To what extent does the body become a central player in defining the politics of epic theatre?

4 Dancing the Wrong Side Out

Archetype in Martha Graham and Jerzy Grotowski

Archetype and the collective unconscious: Carl Gustav Jung's legacy

So far, we have looked at Artaud's notion of the "heart athlete" as it was connected to the human experience of pathos and affect on the basis of our experience of time closely related to dance. Brecht's theatre, on the other hand, emphasized "gestus", the choreographed embodiment of a social constellation, thereby taking a more analytic approach towards the body moving in space. This chapter now explores Carl Gustav Jung's concept of archetype as the body's underlying psychosomatic structure for expression. Dance and theatre of the twentieth century relate to Jung's archetypal psychology, in that both explored the human process of individuation. David Tacey summarizes Jung's impact on the twentieth century, "This was Jung's myth for modernity, offering it something to believe in. God was not dead but had changed his name and location. Salvation had become individuation, the spiritual art of becoming a whole person" (2006, p. 8). For much of the twentieth century, archetypal soul-searching appeared as one of modernity's driving motors explored by a variety of performance practitioners sandwiched between the two world wars. The devastation of the wars left people anxious about human existence as it had been traumatized to the core, when technological development and science were becoming more powerful and life threatening than ever before. This chapter considers how Jungian psychology may inform our engagement with the works of Martha Graham and Jerzy Grotowski to allow for a comparative reading of *Night Journey* (1947/48) and *The Constant Prince* (1965).

Carl Gustav Jung (1875–1961) was a disciple of Sigmund Freud (1856–1939), and both men are recognized as perhaps the two key figures in early twentieth century psychology. With Artaud and the Surrealists they both shared an interest in the unconscious workings of the mind and sought to give an explanation for human behaviour after German philosopher Friedrich Nietzsche (1844–1900) had announced the death of God in his influential *Thus Spoke Zarathustra* (1883–85). The erosion of religious beliefs in the late nineteenth century had a strong impact on Western societies at the time, and early psychology sought to fill this void by exploring the depths of the human mind as the world was on the brink of two disastrous wars. Freud had hoped to access our innermost secrets through the analysis of dreams. He was particularly fascinated by the idea of the unconscious as the realm of our sexual drives and hidden desires which he considered remnants of our instinctual behaviour largely repressed in the course of Western civilization. In his 1930 essay on *Civilization and its Discontents,* Freud characterized our human longing for the sacred as "a sensation of eternity, a feeling as of something limitless, unbounded, something 'oceanic'" (1994, p. 1). Although religious beliefs were increasingly doubted, he still found proof for something mysterious at the heart of human existence as exemplified in our feeling-toned connectedness to nature. The vastness of the ocean serves Freud as the poetic image of felt, core-conscious experience, and Jung later characterized this intuited response as being in tune with the so-called "collective unconscious" (1991). Both Freud and Jung, hence, followed their intuition and became interested to further explore the unconscious mind as an evocative "state of repressed and forgotten contents" (Jung, 1991, p. 3).

The existence of the collective unconscious was a mere hypothesis at its time, and it keeps haunting contemporary neuroscience if we compare it to Damasio's suggestion to think of "proto-consciousness" as the evolutionary forerunner of our minds. More generally, the experience both Jung and Freud were interested to address by this concept is a rather simple one if we simply follow our intuition to ask: Where does our self-consciousness come from before we are born and where does it go, when we die? What happens to our reflective self-awareness during our sleep and what is revealed in our dreams? Perhaps you can make your own experiment and try to remember what it felt like seeing the ocean for the first time: did it affect you in any specific emotional way? You can also observe how many people will stop on the seashore and gaze towards the horizon in a somewhat arrested, dream-state of mind.

Jung was not only interested in the collective unconscious but also the archetypal embodiment of myth and self as can be found in various world religions, literary texts, dreams and media images. But what is an archetype? Although definitions of archetype vary significantly and Jung himself has contributed much to the confusion in the complex and often misunderstood way he was writing, Jung's theories offer an interesting re-evaluation from a postmodern perspective as they question empirical reality and seek for alternatives to Western materialism very much in line with major contemporary concerns over ethics and ecology (Tacey, 2006, p. 115; Stevens, 1994). Departing from Freud's original idea of repression, Jung believed in a wider concept of the unconscious suggesting that our mind could be separated into a personal (derived from our life experience and toned by our feelings) and transpersonal dimension (universal structure). Jung's depth psychology thus seeks to amplify our individual dream images by relating them to myths and symbols as they occur in all cultures at all times (Tacey, 2006, p. 4). It is particularly interesting to note that he emphasizes how art and creativity often derive from an intuitive force rather than conscious process and we will see how both Graham's and Grotowski's physical training prepare their performers to access such intuition on the level of impulse and energy.

Considering the significance of myth in human experience, Jung suggests that it provides us with a language that expresses our "unconscious psychic process" (1991, p. 6). Myth and the collective unconscious form the realm of Jung's so-called archetypes. According to Jung, such archetypal figures are the mother, the child, the trickster, the wise old man, the hero, the fool, the devil, the temptress, the scapegoat, the healer and ultimately also our much cherished idea of self. To take the mother archetype as an example, we can think of our own mother, who we may share a very personal relationship with, and the cultural archetype of motherhood traditionally defined as caring, protective, loving, etc. Jung regarded these latter qualities as archetypal, because women may become such mothers everywhere in the world, although uncaring, cold and unloving mothers may also exist. Archetypal images are therefore often intuitively understood although fundamentally changeable, as Jung explains,

> The fact is that archetypal images are so packed with meaning in themselves that people never think of asking what they really do mean. That the gods die from time to time is due to man's sudden discovery that they do not mean anything, that they are made by human hands, useless idols of wood and stone. In reality, however, he has merely discovered that up till then he has never thought about his images at all. And when he starts thinking about them, he does so with the help of what he calls "reason" – which in point of fact is nothing more than the sum-total of all his prejudices and myopic views. (1991, pp. 12–13)

One of the most interesting aspects for our study of the body in this context, however, is Jung's archetypal study of the individuation process and its relationship to the self in performance. Jung defines the capital letter Self as the archetype of archetypes which we have to be careful not to confuse with the small letter self that refers to the person, or ego in Freud's theory of the modern subject so very influential for Western conceptions of individualism (Stevens, 1994, pp. 33–34). The cosmological Self is universal consciousness as embodied in various manifestations including the natural environment, animal life and human existence. Sherry Salman's reading of Jung is helpful to understand the relevance of the archetypal Self at the heart of our embodied life experience as it allows human perception to relate and engage with the world. She suggests that we consider archetype as a given psychosomatic structure "from a time when consciousness did not think, but only perceived" (Jung, 1991, p. 33).

Her perspective on Jung's theories may easily be aligned with the already mentioned shift towards phenomenology and experience in the early twentieth century. Archetypal structures are hence – just like Damasio's emphasis on emotion and core-consciousness or Bergson's notion of soul – at the heart of the meaning making process and allow us to mediate our perception of inner and outer worlds. Salman defines,

> As psychosomatic "structures", they [archetypes] are our innate capacity to apprehend, organize, and create experience. Archetypes are both biologically based patterns of behaviour and the symbolic images of these patterns. As transpersonal structures, they are transcendental "essences" or quintessential distillates of imagination and meaning. Archetypes, with their ties to both subject and object,

> unfold simultaneously in both radical specificity and subjectivity (the intrapsychic, symbolic dimension), and in numerous embodied avenues of experience and expression, as living mythologems. (2008, p. 63)

From a phenomenological perspective archetypes may thus be defined as "categories of imagination" and our "innate possibilities of ideas" rather than the ideas themselves (Adams, 2008, p. 108). This distinction is very important to recognize, for often popular discourse confounds archetype for what is actually stereotype. However, whereas stereotype is merely constructed on the discursive level of concept, an archetype has a much deeper, experiential and psycho-somatic relationship to embodiment and evolutionary memory. More contemporary definitions of archetype thus acknowledge its relation to the personal context and suggest that archetypes are merely universal on a structural level that is shaping human consciousness rather than universal per se. To conclude, we can assert that archetypes reside in the deeper layers of our psycho-somatic awareness and experience of the world which means that they allow us to construct inner and outer images of the world in a meaningful way.

Following this post-Jungian analysis of archetype as psycho-somatic structure, we can now turn towards the archetypal analysis of twentieth-century theatre and dance as it opens up a perspective from which we can gain deeper insights into the relationship between embodiment, experience and the creative process. In this chapter, we focus on Martha Graham and Jerzy Grotowski who had both read Jung, and archetype appears as a strong creative force in their distinct works. Their use of archetypal s/Self-exploration in dance and theatre is interesting for us to examine as they both demonstrate how the embodied investment in myth becomes a performative strategy that writes dance into twentieth-century Western theatre forms and ultimately transforms Western conceptions of corporeality and identity thereafter.

Martha Graham (1894–1991)

A contemporary to Brecht and Artaud – just that she lived much longer – Martha Graham is considered one of the most important modern dance choreographers of the twentieth century. Alongside several other women pioneers of American modern dance of the early twentieth century, for example Isadora Duncan and Ruth St Denis, she rebelled against confined ideals of the nineteenth-century corset-girded female body. "Movement never lies", her father had explained, when Graham was still a young girl in unrivalled admiration of his work as a doctor in early psychiatry (Graham, 1991, p. 20). She became interested in the workings of the human soul, as expressed in our daily movements, ever since. Martha Graham's career as a dancer and choreographer followed her father's initial idea, and many of her dances express the psychological turmoil of the first half of the twentieth century. Martha Graham conceives of the soul as our "inner landscape" (1991, p. 4), when she explains,

> It is through this that the legends of the soul's journey are retold with all their tragedy and their bitterness and sweetness of living. It is at this point that the sweep of life catches up with the mere personality of the performer, and while the individual becomes greater, the personal becomes less personal. And there is grace. I mean the grace resulting from faith ... faith in life, in love, in people, in the act of dancing. (1991, p. 5)

We can see from this quote that Graham shared Jung's interest in myth and archetype as much as the idea of the unconscious as the realm of our emotional worlds. Jung explained our desire to express such inner landscapes as the modernist quest for "effective images, the thought-forms that satisfy the restlessness of heart and mind" to conquer fears of nihilism in the wake of rationalism and religious doubt (1991, p. 14). Archetypes are therefore precisely such primal "thought forms" which allow for our meaningful experience of the world, inter-human relationships and natural environment. This notion of the archetypal thought-image will be useful, when we analyse how Martha Graham worked with archetype in her choreography of *Night Journey*.

In praise of female creativity: Martha Graham's *Night Journey* (1947), filmed 1961

Martha Graham's *Night Journey* (1947) delves into the psycho-poetic depths of the Oedipus myth. In developing the choreography, Graham focused on the fate of Jocasta, the neglected heroine of the classical

Greek drama by Sophocles. Her departure point for investigating the Oedipus myth was taken from Greek tragedy as the programme notes and prologue to the film testify, although she subsequently reframed the choreographic narrative by focusing on the female perspective for her dance. Hence, quite unlike Sophocles, Martha Graham was not that much interested in the male protagonist of the ancient tragedy, but she identified with Jocasta, the female tragic heroine, of the play. Whereas most of the history of Western theatre, psychology and philosophy has been obsessed with Oedipus as the incestuous "figurehead of imperialism" (Foucault, 1972, p. xx), Graham composes a dance choreography that places Jocasta's emotional torment at the centre of the unfolding action. As outlined by the original programme notes,

> This dance is a legend of recognition. The action takes place in Jocasta's heart at the moment when she recognizes the ultimate terms of her destiny. She enters her room when the precise fulfilment of its terms awaits her. Here the Daughters of Night, Oedipus in his inescapable role, and the Seer pursue themselves across her heart in that instant of agony. (Reprinted in: Morris, 2001, p. 67)

Martha Graham's choreography makes "that instant of agony" the starting point of her dance exploration, while the actions "pursue themselves across her heart" (Morris, 2001, p. 67). Down to the very choice of wording Graham evokes the Artaudian notion of the "heart athlete" and musical tempo of "passionate time" to guide her into the psychological dreamwork her dance involves. The costume, make-up and minimal props allow her for an associative object transformation to embody Jocasta's primal fate as her own. Thus, *Night Journey*'s cathartic climax does not culminate in Oedipus' blindness, but Jocasta's suicide. She kills herself, because she cannot bear to be the wife and mother to the abhorrent figure of imperialism she has birthed.

Critics have commented on her difficult relationship to Erick Hawkins at the time, an attractive and significantly younger dancer who became Graham's lover and later husband to then compete with her for company leadership (see Franko, 2012). Graham's dance hence unfolds in response to pathos, desire and in its intricate relationship to power. In the film version Bertram Ross becomes the object of the female erotic gaze, his pelvis surrounded by golden ornaments in similar shape to Graham's snake brooch on her breasts, a symbol of provocative attraction, youth and fertility. He appears as the archetypal hero and lover, master and child in relationship to Graham, who is anything but a weak woman. Although ballet vocabulary was becoming more evident in Graham's choreographies of the 1940s (see Bannerman, 1999), no one could be farther from the romantic ballerina than the already elderly Graham in her powerful poise dancing for the 1961 film version. Hence, Graham's aesthetic is less of an imitation of narrative ballet than a precursor of dance theatre. The dance has been interpreted as a woman's coming-of-age in the second half of the twentieth century (compare Burt, 1998, Bannerman, 2010). Graham did not have any children herself but chose the profession; she was sexually assertive, but not easily exploited; and we can see all of that life experience expressed in her forceful movement vocabulary at the advanced age of sixty-five.

The 1961 film version begins with a close up of Isamu Noguchi's set, before the camera turns sideways and reveals Jocasta, alias Martha Graham. Unmistakably, *Night Journey* presents the audience with the mindscape of Jocasta's inner world as revealed by the embodiment of the myth. As we know from her notebook as well as her collaboration with her set designer Isamu Noguchi, both the set and the roles of the other dancers evolved as extensions of Graham's physical anatomy. In that sense, she used the sculptural element as a "gesturely tool" (Noguchi, 1986, p. 10). As Noguchi further explained,

> The man and woman, or Oedipus and Jocasta, are there in my bed but in the most rudimentary sense. These are not human beings. They are effigies. [...] Martha often says, "I need a place to sit", a woman's place or a bed. [...] When I had to make a woman's place, I made a seat shaped as an hourglass. [...] The seat is an extension of your spine. (Tracy, 1986, p. 14)

The significance of the bed as symbol of sleep, matrimony and childbirth makes the dream structure sculpturally evident and aligns the Jungian idea of amplification with the legend's dramaturgy of recognition. Genevieve Oswald refers to the treatment of time as represented in the symbolic meaning of the bed as an hourglass:

> In "Night Journey" the woman's place, Jocasta's place, the Queen's place or the royal place, is a stool fashioned in the shape of an hourglass. To Noguchi the designer, it is a symbol of woman's figure; but

> it is also symbol of the time of night, the hourglass, is the god of darkness as her lover, so the use of the symbol of the time of night, the hourglass, is appropriate. (1983, p. 46)

Furthermore, Oswald's interpretation of the dance points out that Martha Graham's interest in the myth focused on Jocasta as a mother archetype symbolized by the "intertwined serpents forming the brooch on her breast and the ornament in her hair" (1985, p. 45).

There is a severe archetypal reverence that Graham pays tribute to as she dresses up in front of the mirror evoking the myth of Jocasta as part of her process of transformation. Although the seriousness she displays in the film appears somewhat of a parody for our contemporary sensibility, it testifies to the psychological dimension carried further by her exploration of myth and archetype in dance. As Mark Franko has argued, the archetypal confrontation created a "monstrous body" in the sense that Graham's performance became larger than life by "encrypting" haunting psychological truths of times past and present (2012, pp. 61–62). He explains how the dance referenced repressed psychological and mythical content that audiences related to as they became active collaborators (2012, p. 8). Not unlike the spectators in Brecht's 1949 production of *Mother Courage*, Graham's audiences also related to the gestic impact of her dance as much as they responded to the spatial choreography. As Franko comments, dance for Graham was about "showing" emotional content as a condensation of time and space as present-centred affectedness, whereas choreography was to "tell" the narrative of the dance and therefore slightly less important in its mere dramaturgical function (2012, pp. 104–105).

Graham was already in her mid-sixties, when *A Dancer's World* was produced and much of her commentary appeared as part of her legacy to the dance world (see Acocella, 2009). In the film *A Dancer's World* (1957) Graham comments on the creative process of how costume and make-up help her transform and find the character looking back at her in the mirror, but how it is ultimately the physical work in the studio that prepares her for the part. As a result, Martha Graham's belief that "dance is communication" that expresses the "deep matters of the heart" speaks of the feeling-toned, phenomenological sensibility of her work, although much of her actual dance vocabulary includes habitual everyday movement (see "A Dancer's World", 1957). In a way, we may say that her dances synchronize affect and gestus as explored in the works and writings of Artaud and Brecht previously. Gay Morris thus points towards "the possibility of dance ordering thoughts and feelings not just through choreography but in the basic techniques of comportment that present the body to the world" (2001, p. 57). Graham herself comments on the importance of practice in the studio as the founding preparation for her dance, when she says,

> I believe that we learn by practice. Whether it means to learn to dance by practicing dancing or to learn to live by practicing living, the principles are the same. In each it is the performance of a dedicated precise set of acts, physical or intellectual, from which comes shape of achievement, a sense of one's being, a satisfaction of spirit. One becomes in some area an athlete of God. (1991, p. 3)

For Martha Graham her dance was thus intricately bound up with her life, and practice evolved from letting her life inform the dance and vice versa.

Graham technique

In the prologue section of the film *A Dancer's World,* Martha Graham explains how her technique prepares the dancer's body as a fully responsive instrument through which he or she can express herself. As explained above, Graham was most interested in the inner workings of our psyche and all of her dances explored some of the deeper conflicts from our emotional experience of the world. Martha Graham believed that our body is a perfect index of such feelings and that we can communicate these in dance. Important elements of her technique to convey this are contract/release and the spiral, movement processes which recur throughout the various floor exercises, standing positions and travelling movements. However, the extent to which Eastern yogic practices influenced American modern dance should also be noticed. As Horosko has pointed out,

> This ancient awareness of the physicality of movement as dependent on the breath, and the anatomical changes in the body due to the breathing process, was based on her early training in Eastern dance forms in the Denishawn Company. Although yogalike breathing was

> introduced into the classrooms of Western dance at the turn of the century, Graham was the first to develop breath with the contraction and release principle into an inherent basis of movement in her new dance form. (Horosko, 1991, p. x)

This allowed Graham a much deeper exploration of the anatomy and physiology underlying the mobilization of the pelvis and breathing into the lower spine as the seat of sexual–creative energy. As Horosko further describes,

> It was the first time [1927–28] that Martha used the terms contraction and release as an awareness of a whole new approach to the physicality of movement dependent upon the breath and the anatomical changes in the body due to the breathing process. It was this awareness of the changes of the body due to breathing in and breathing out that freed Martha Graham from her Denishawn ethnic influence as well as the ballet influence. She had found a way to create her own dances, using the contraction and release principle. She found the answer to her own need to discover and explore what the body could do. (2002, p. 21)

In her recent book *Vagina. A New Biography* (2012), Naomi Wolf delivers the neurophysiological evidence that connects female orgasm to women's creativity – a truth Martha Graham had most certainly discovered for herself in breathing and contracting deeply in the sacred centre of her pelvis, a technique derived from her introduction to yoga via the orientalist appropriation by Denishawn and Ruth St. Denis (see Srinivasan, 2012). As early as 1948 she thus attempted to right a Western wrong that cast female sexuality in the shadow of male domination and fulfilment. Diving into the emotional depth of one's own body connected her dancers to an archetypal level of identification with the mythic depths of female creativity expressed through dance by emphasizing the importance of her breathing technique. Horosko explains,

> Martha wanted to give us the feeling of the depth of movement. We were not to be two-dimensional. We had to feel the inner skeleton of the body as part of the whole movement. The deep dramatic quality came on the exhalation of breath, or the contraction; the lyric and open quality on the inhalation of the breath, or the release. (2002, p. 23)

We can see some of the evidence in *A Dancer's World*, although the camera takes away much of the energetic field and overt eroticism that would have surrounded the live performance. Nonetheless, Graham's firm belief in the relationship between body and soul convinced her that the dancer through the exact exploration of breath and movement can access an archetypal truthfulness that transcends the actual autobiographical self of the performer. Her representation of Jocasta thus embodied archetypal facets of female experience – love, birth and death – across time. Susan Foster, on the other hand, has emphasized the Freudian repression of sexual desires and emotional needs conveyed by her work suggesting that

> The self is too dark and repressed, the act of expression too tortured for movement to be light and free-flowing. The ideal body, then, even as it manifests an agile responsiveness, also shows in the strained quality and definition of its musculature the ordeal of expression. (1997, p. 245)

The samples of Graham technique from *A Dancer's World* demonstrate how the technique emphasizes strength, flexibility and endurance. While these qualities clearly stand out, they are also a remarkable testimony to a woman's feisty creativity as she contested the legacy of paternalistic hegemony and fascism (see Franko, 2012, p. 90). At the same time, the emphasis on pelvic floor work and the contraction as the energetic source of outward propelling movement asserted female sexuality as a means to approach a holistic sense of self and empowerment for men and women alike. As Henrietta Bannerman's insightful analysis of female empowerment in Graham's work concludes,

> The contraction is housed in the pelvic area, which for Graham dancers, male and female alike, is the well-spring or core of physical energy. For women this is the center of femaleness, and for Graham it was both the source of all genuine movement and bodily gesture, which, as we have seen, within the context of her range of dances, is an energy that is molded into a formalized method of expressing the intangible and the sensory. (2010, pp. 41–43)

Graham's *Night Journey* thus provides us with a remarkable testimony to women's liberation during the twentieth century making the female

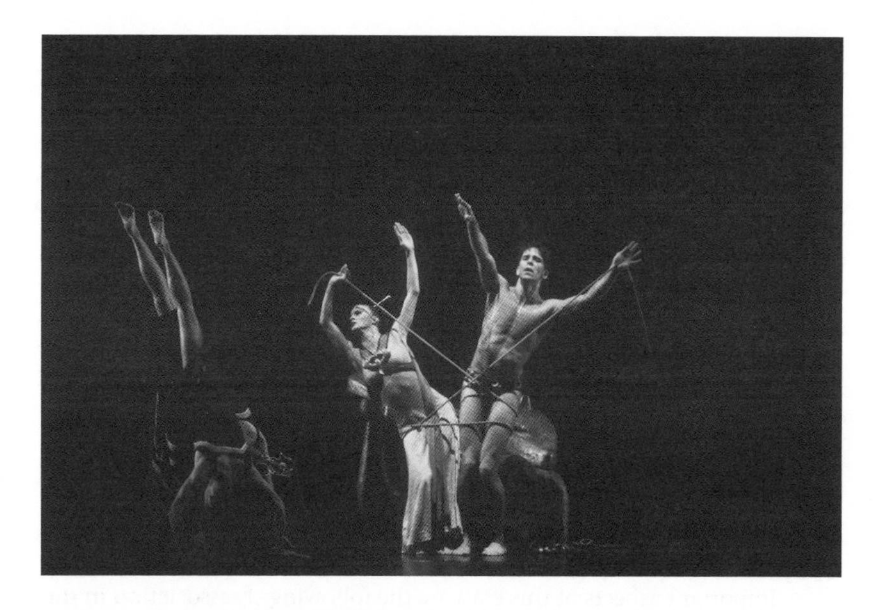

Terese Capucilli, Kenneth Topping (on rock) and Pascal Rioult in Martha Graham's *Night Journey* © Nan Melville.

body the centre of her anatomic explorations and choreography. Her archetypal explorations of myth are based in a core-conscious exploration of the interrelationship between movement, breath and feeling paired with the habitual gestures of everyday movements and gendered codifications. In many ways, her dance is theatre as much as her theatre is dance. She is therefore one of the pioneers of the hybrid genre called dance theatre, which will be discussed in more detail later.

Jerzy Grotowski (1933–1999)

Jerzy Grotowski's *Towards a Poor Theatre* (1991) first published in 1968, is probably one of the most cited key texts for performance in the twentieth century, which influenced many of the other directors and even choreographers discussed in this book. The theme of this revolutionary book was the idea of poor theatre itself. What does it mean? Grotowski's call for a poor theatre suggests that we have to do away with spectacle in the theatre, including such elements as scenery, lighting, props, music and several other embellishments of the nineteenth-century realist convention as to arrive at the simple relationship between actors and the audience. Before Jerzy Grotowski became a theatre director he had been trained as an actor and was influenced by Stanislavsky's work on physical actions, yet for Grotowski working on physical actions was primarily concerned with the eradication and elimination of psychic blocks.

Grotowski thus refers to the actor's performance as a total gift which means that the actor's job is not so much to imitate the character, but to reveal his or her own inner truth. For that she needs to undertake rigorous training which in many ways becomes a kind of research encounter with the archetypal layers of our conscious mind as the source of theatrical expression. As one can see, there is a sense of discipline and craft similar to dance in the actor training that is the basis for Grotowski's approach which attempts to confront the actor's inner psychological blocks to arrive at a mature state of full expressivity and creative potential.

Important aspects of this craft are the following: 1. association in the form of a physical reaction of memory, 2. impulse as a "reaction that begins inside the body and which is visible only when it has already become a small action" (Richards, 1995, p. 94), 3. scoring as the "fixing of moments of contact between you and your partner(s)" (Slowiak and Cuesta, 2007, p. 65) and 4. contact as "being present" in a combination of seeing, listening and responding in the moment. The performer should strive for signs that derive from pure impulses and avoid realistic clichés. Grotowski said that the body has its own way of remembering; indeed, he believed with Bergson, Jung, Artaud and Graham that the body is memory with all our evolutionary baggage stored in the psychosomatic structure of our spine and autonomous nervous system.

Unlike Stanislavski's early work in acting which suggested that the character emerges from an associative experience based in the actor's real life, Grotowski proposed that we do not so much need to remember the feeling itself, but can actually rely on the physical actions to create emotion in the first place. Grotowski would claim the body remembers what it was doing at the time, rather than what it was feeling, and thus he somewhat reversed the logic of those theatre and dance practitioners before him. To create poor theatre, all the precise details of a movement are therefore important to recall, likewise all the impulses and energies that reveal the inner landscapes of our being (Slowiak and Cuesta, 2007, p. 68).

Theatre in the state of grace – Jerzy Grotwoski's *The Constant Prince* (1965)

Based on the 2005 digital reconstruction of *The Constant Prince* by Ferrucio Marotti held by the Grotowski Archive at University of Kent, the following analysis examines Grotowski's confrontation with the Christ archetype by focusing on Ryszard Cieślak's performance as Constant Prince. Cieślak's legendary performance recreated the Prince's martyrdom as a contemporary allegory of suffering and perseverance under occupation not unlike the situation of Poland between Nazi Germany and Communist Russia. On the archetypal level, his performance's gift was not unlike that of Christ, an act of self-sacrificing love and redemption. Dressed in the iconic white shirt and loincloth that Ryszard Cieślak came to be remembered by, his performance became an allegory of the human condition.

Early on in the film version the performers surround Cieślak whose body is stretched apparently lifeless across a table which presents an image reminiscent of T. S. Eliot's "patient etherised upon a table" from one of the twentieth century's most iconic modernist poems *The Lovesong of J. Alfred Prufrock*. The performers check Cieślak's pulse, listen to his fluttering heart beat gestured through Mirecka's elbow rising and falling frantically and utter poetically sounding but barely recognizable words expressing "longing", "sadness" and "captivity". Barely audible, there is also mention of a life measured by "heart aches" and "pain" with time as "master of the world [...] and the soul's grief" (00:00:15:21-00:01:59:22). While the dramatic text almost disappears during this scene, the movement score could not have made its meaning more transparent as the performers gather around the table in a state of loss and confusion mourning the seemingly dead Cieślak as Constant Prince. All that remains clear from the evidence of the visual documentation is the state of loss these characters convey: Phenix questions her beauty as it belies her tormented soul and can no longer recognize her image in the mirror or praise the beauty of the garden outside or the melancholy sunset over the sea. Similarly, the stallion's power – as that of the ancient god Helios – is defeated by thoughts of powerlessness and inner injury (00:02:16:19-00:03:02:07).

Tellingly, the performance opens with the prologue to Calderón's *Great Theatre of the World*, when Mirecka gestures the emasculation of the performer who is dressed in the costume for his performance of

Don Enrique. Phenix, on the other hand, holds on to her "deep sorrow" which she clings to like the white shirt in her hands symbolizing the loss of innocence as upon the return of her lover Muléy, she will be married off to the Infant of Morocco in the following scene. Her sorrow is the mirror image to the martyrdom of Don Fernando (Ryszard Cieślak), the Constant Prince, who now enters wrapped in a glaring red cloth.

The cuts of the original text juxtapose the exchange between Phenix and Muléy, who fight over their worldly love betrayed as they argue over jealousy and pain. The play debates worldly power and whether one needs to obey the king or follow one's own faith. A split of consciousness occurs at the heart of the play's misery and melancholy tone when Phenix picks up the red cloth to look at Don Fernando's face as she says, "Ah, what a sad moment ... Ah, how this sad miniature is looking at me!" (00:08:50:16-00:08:55:16). The King – as the representation of worldly power politics –meanwhile diverts himself by playing his cruel fights as he deals his slaves yet another card or role to play and treats them well ("in your hands there are no end of favours"). And yet he is a "savage lord" as he makes his slaves "forget their fatherland" and doubt their faith. Clearly, this could be Poland under Russian Communism. Thus the chorus of fascist supporters carry Don Fernando on their shoulders – not unlike Judases they lift him up – to let him fall into death and despair alone.

And yet, the play must go on: "Sing slaves". One more time, the chorus examines the Prince's body, his life functions and reflexes, the beating heart like a fluttering bird's wing. Still Phenix cannot recognize her face in the mirror, for all its beauty there is no essence to her appearance. Then, the ritualistic transformation begins as the chorus sings and builds up to the Prince's god-like trance and allegorical crucifixion that transcends human suffering in the act of faithful love. Ryszard Cieślak's first monologue sets up his total act of deliverance and glorious illumination (00:16:33:06-00:19:29:20). Even on the tape he stands out as a possessed man, shaking ecstatically as the words tumble out of his mouth and exhausted body, trembling through the end of his lines. Meanwhile the chorus walks around in circles, supporting his trance with their feet drumming the rhythm.

Grotowski's script for the performance reworked Calderón's text as a montage that kept a fraction of archetypal motifs which became important in the collective creation of the final performance work. Not unlike Martha Graham's confrontation of the Oedipus myth, Grotowski, too, chose a contemporary perspective as his point of departure by asking:

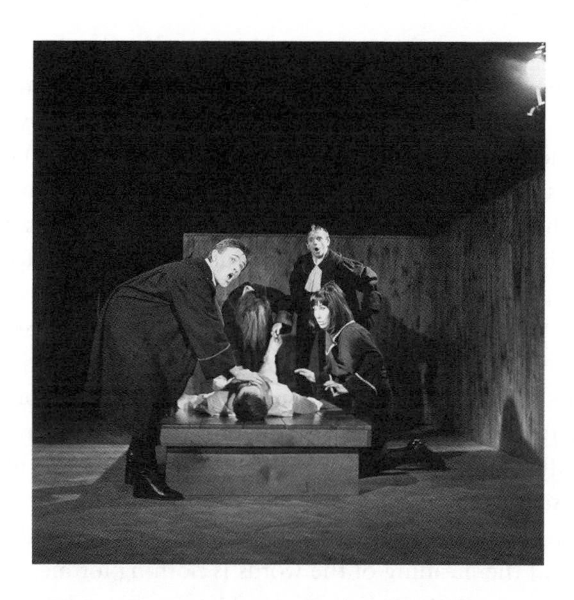

***The Constant Prince*, version I; Wrocław 1965; Mieczysław Janowski, Maja Komorowska, Antoni Jahołkowski, Rena Mirecka and Ryszard Cieślak © Photo of Laboratory Theatre.**

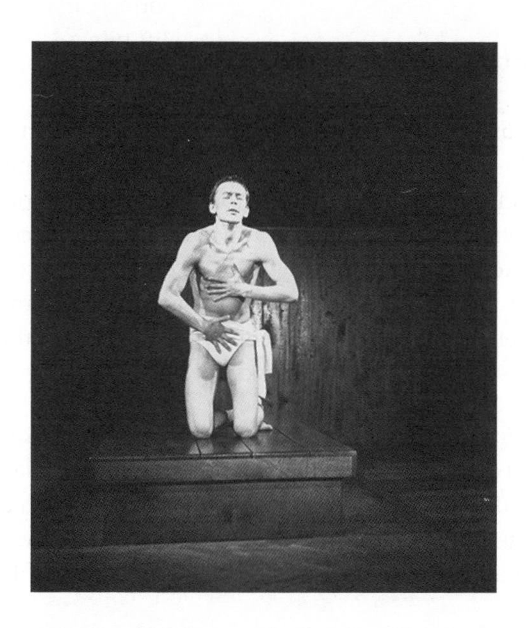

***The Constant Prince*, version I; Wrocław 1965; Ryszard Cieślak © Photo of Laboratory Theatre.**

What does the myth say to us now? How do we relate to its archetypal patterns from our own inner sources of movement and creativity?

Tellingly, theatre critic Bentley (1969) referred to *The Constant Prince* as a "one-act dance drama" (p. 169, quoted in Slowiak, 2007, p. 90). Grotowski's approach was dialectical in the sense that he built opposition into the structure of his performance work. Acting was not about finding a character but revealing one's true self as opposed to the roles actors play as persons in their everyday lives (Slowiak and Cuesta, 2007, p. 94). Grotowski refers to this process as "total acceptance" of one's self and one's myth – finding one's own Christ or Jocasta buried deep in the psycho-somatic patterns of our archetypal wiring that connects our body's energy centres to our archaic brain memory. As Zygmunt Molik explains, this approach emphasizes a phenomenology of life, where the expression of a fully embodied energetic understanding supersedes the meaning of words. Molik comments in conversation with Guiliano Campo: "[...] the meaning of the words is nothing for me, something else is important: what Life is given, the Life the person brings out with these words. What sound, what feelings with this sound. The meaning of the words is the last thing; it isn't my problem" (2010, p. 17).

Jerzy Grotowski: Performer training

In the famous essay "From the Theatre Company to Art as Vehicle" Grotowski introduced the term "craft" as a relevant concept of performer training which prepared the actor's body through song, impulse, forms of movement and textual motifs to create what later came to be known as "Action" (Richards, 1995, p. 122). The treatise introduced a major shift from theatre for audiences towards a performative theatre of experience and self, a therapeutic process "toward the essential" (Richards, 1995, p. 124). As Grotowski explains,

> Art as vehicle is like a very primitive elevator: it's some kind of basket pulled by a cord, with which the doer lifts himself toward a more subtle energy, to descend with this to the instinctual body. This is the objectivity of the ritual. If Art as vehicle functions, this objectivity exists and the basket moves for those who do the Action. (Richards, 1995, p. 125)

This release of energy and impulse connects performers on a self-transformative level which is on the verge of therapy and healing – "a living hymn to human existence" as embodied in Ryszard Cieslak's ecstatic performance in *The Constant Prince*:

> Finally he becomes a living hymn in homage to human existence, in spite of his having been persecuted and stupidly humiliated. The Prince's ecstasy is his suffering which he can endure only by offering himself to the truth as if in an act of love. (Grotowski, 1991, p. 82–83)

Grotowski's approach to Calderón's text was therefore more interested in the abstract theme or motif than the literal dramatization. As Slowiak points out, Grotowski's approach towards the text was a deconstruction to reveal the text's significance for contemporary times and audiences. Using Meyerhold's principle of choreographic montage, the dramatic text was reworked so that the actor can explore him- or herself within it (Slowiak and Cuesta, 2007, p. 15). While such emancipation could be guaranteed in the face-to-face encounter during the rehearsal process, such engagement was almost impossible to achieve on behalf of the audiences. And yet, the spectator was carefully cast in each production to maximize a participatory function in the event (Slowiak and Cuesta, 2007, p. 17). Grotowski emphasized craft as a form of spiritual work on oneself, not unlike ancient techniques of mysticism (Slowiak and Cuesta, 2007, p. 19).

This may be achieved in the trance-like state of what Grotowski called "translumination" (Slowiak and Cuesta, 2007, pp. 60–61). Translumination or trance are terms connected to the emergence of a different consciousness, as a perceivable manifestation of changing energy, and are derived from the precise repetition of the acting score. Grotowski integrated forms from Haitian *yanvalou* dance in order to teach actors how to access primary levels of energy – those that Zygmunt Molik referred to as "The Life"– derived from movements originating in the lower spine. As a precise technique of ritual, this allows for harmonious improvisation as it provides a structure from within which the performer can become free in his or her exploration of movement and expression. Similar to how the form serves the dissolution of the self in Haitian *vodou*, where the dancer embodies *damballah* the snake god, it also serves Grotowski as a means to connect to a source of animation and tradition. He claims,

> One access to the creative way consists of discovering in yourself an ancient corporality to which you are bound by a strong ancestral

> relation. So you are neither in the character nor in the non-character. Starting from details you can discover in you somebody other – your grandfather, your mother. (Slowiak and Cuesta, 2007, p. 82)

Authenticity thus emerges from the body as the performer's memory, life, and essence (see Slowiak and Cuesta, 2007, p. 68).

What Grotowski describes as essence, and interpreted by Slowiak and Cuesta to refer to the performer's quest of self, may in Jungian terms be described as a quest for the Self as the embodiment of a fuller cosmological consciousness unleashing an experience of flow embedded in the mind's circular relationship that transitions between self and void (see Csikszentmihalyi, 2002, pp. 34–35). As with flow experiences in general – such as those while enjoying a good run, sex or night out partying – here too, time is suspended in an instant of duration where our awareness of past and present are merged. This implies that body memory is activated through creativity and is potentially therapeutic in our coming to terms with ourselves as the compound of all our memories, ideas, desires and actions experienced.

Essence may thus be defined as the core-conscious impulse that bypasses social conditioning and creates a physical expression to build an organic movement score for performance. Such scoring is initially improvised but can be fixed by those physically remembered actions. Grotowski's approach towards movement is therefore not unlike dance improvisation in that he explores the source of creativity based in the spinal cord and its different energy centres of the body and autonomous nervous system. And he even claims, "At a moment of psychic shock, a moment of terror, of mortal danger or tremendous joy, a man does not behave 'naturally'. A man in an elevated spiritual state uses rhythmically articulated signs, begins to dance, to sing" (1991, pp. 17–18). Such movement energy connects to our unconscious, archetypal impulses, and memories. Indeed, Grotowski's exploration of Haitian *yanvalou* dance later in his career testifies to this as his exploration looked for the mystical link between embodiment and spirituality, similar to Graham's discoveries via yoga. In that sense, Grotowski brings theatre closer to dance by training his performers to access the organic Life source. In his search for a more truthful experience of human existence, Grotowski refers to this situation as a "space where one does not lie to oneself, that which we do is what it is and we do not pretend it is anything else" (Osiński, 1986, p. 123).

Material derived from physical movement improvisation was written down in notebooks, where performers differentiated between their actions and associations. As this material was discussed and reconstructed, the score emerged from the key elements that make up the signs which again are based on living impulses (Slowiak and Cuesta, 2007, pp. 88–89). The script was reworked as a montage, and the text remained an important element in the collective creation of the final performance work. Grotowski's approach was dialectical in the sense that he built opposition into the structure of his performance work. Acting was not about finding a character modelled on everyday life but rather to reveal one's true self by confronting the core-conscious archetype (Slowiak and Cuesta, 2007, p. 94).

The social mask: Pierre Bourdieu's concept of habitus

Grotowski considered this work important in order to allow the actor to break away from what he referred to as the "social mask" (1991). He believed that the social mask hides our true being from the world. While it allows us to perform according to certain social conventions – being a good student, loving husband, mother, wife, teacher, etc. – it does not account for the complexity of our psyches and inner worlds. Grotowski suggests that we need to find expression that is closer to dance or singing to embody our true joys and anxieties. This is an interesting idea, which we also find in sociology, where the French sociologist Pierre Bourdieu (1930–2002) has coined the analogous term "habitus" (1977).

Pierre Bourdieu's concept of habitus is quite similar to Grotowski's notion of the social mask or Brecht's gestus for that matter and helps us to better understand what this term means in relationship to Grotowski's theatre and the actor's task. In sociology, habitus characterizes all patterns of human behaviour: the way we move, put up our hair, glance at each other, etc. Bourdieu suggests that there are certain rules we learn to be successfully integrated into social life. Most of these rules are learnt quite early, when we are children. For example, how to use the toilet, how to use the knife and fork for eating, etc. Since we repeat these actions everyday, they become part of our daily routine, something which Bourdieu refers to as "practical faith" (1977), because we no longer think about doing any of this – we just do it. In that sense habitus is pre-reflective, because we no longer think about how we do certain things, we take this behaviour for granted and it also reassures us of our own social identity as members of a certain group, a family, a sports team or a class. Habitus becomes our second nature – who we represent in society – and thereby functions as symbolic capital that we exchange for respect, acceptance and social integration (Bourdieu, 1977, pp. 72–95). Social habitus, however, limits or confines our means of expressing ourselves creatively as its routine everyday performances go unquestioned. While habitus protects our inner self, Grotowski challenges his actors to move beyond their habitual comfort zone by removing that layer of the socialization process. The act of transition whereby the actor removes the social mask and reveals an inner truth transforms her into what Grotowski has termed the "holy actor" (1991) – a performer who creates from the sacred centre and mobilizes all her energy levels. Such performance is very focused and present in the here and now – totally giving as an act of self-deliverance.

Technically, the actor achieves this state by confronting the myth or archetype - to use the Jungian term - of the dramatic text. However, unlike Stanislavski's earlier approach, one does not simply identify and imitate the archetypal structure but rather confronts and works through its deeper psychological layer. As our mind contains the whole of the archetypal set-up, a performer taps into the depth of her inner soul to resurface as a transformed human being at the completion of this process which, however, may be a life's work. Such confrontation needs to consider the contemporary moment, because we no longer believe in the same systems and themes as generations before us. Working in confrontation with the archetypal myth the performer trains the body to develop a sense of technique and discipline to undertake her research on physical actions. One of the techniques that Grotowski effectively introduced was using the vocal resonators in the body by singing the so-called songs of tradition, as well as by the physical manipulation of different energy levels as they emerge from using impulse in physical actions which were then determined by a fixed movement score, similar to the ritualistic performance in mysticism or yogic practice.

Grotowski's training thus prepares the body to enter a state of heightened physical awareness which allows the performer to deliver the total act whereby performers are open – somewhat radiant – in their response to each other but also in their direct communication with the audience.

Grotowski describes this as "struggle with one's own truth" in the following quote from *Towards a Poor Theatre*:

> In this struggle with one's own truth, this effort to peel off the life-mask, the theatre, with its full-fleshed perceptivity, has always seemed to me a place of provocation. It is capable of challenging itself and its audience by violating accepted stereotypes of vision, feeling, and judgement – more jarring because it is imaged in human organism's breath, body, and inner impulses. This defiance of taboo, this transgression, provides the shock which rips off the mask, enabling us to give ourselves nakedly to something which is impossible to define but which contains Eros and Caritas. (1991, pp. 21–22)

Historically, we may argue that Grotowski's work with the actor developed a psycho-somatically oriented form of psychotherapy to redress some of the traumatic effects of coming to terms with the horrors of the stifling effects of the Second World War on his generation. Eros and Caritas are the two archetypal principles derived from the teachings of Christ: love and compassion. The physical process develops stamina in the actor: a way of caring and loving the physical work is necessary to gain the confidence that allows the performer to not only engage openly with herself but also with her partner and audience. Buried under layers of civilization and trauma, however, those ancient techniques – still very much present in South Asian, African and Caribbean performance cultures today – had to be relearnt by actors in the West. Layers of social masking had to be peeled away to reconnect body and mind structures on a deeper spiritual level. The actor's epiphany then is but a mere recognition of her self-worth and creativity: the will to affirm her own life as the sacred core of existence.

Paratheatre: Moving towards life

Paratheatre, as it evolved from Grotowski's work with the actor, was concerned with the process of creativity and created what is conceptualized as active culture where a sense of companionship involved all participants in the act (Slowiak and Cuesta, 2007, p. 34). It was strictly life affirming in its opposition to deathly politics that surrounded Grotowski's generation that was moving from the horrors of fascism, to communism and the war in Vietnam. Paratheatre taught participants in the experiment to move beyond ego-consciousness, however, it held no techniques on how to integrate these powerful experiences of blissful ecstatic existence in everyday life. As Slowiak and Cuesta critically observed, "reintegration" was not part of the teachings, and participants were oftentimes left alone with ensuing depression and helplessness (2007, p. 39). Grotowski's late experiments in transculturalism concerned themselves with the search for a theatre of sources focusing on simple physical actions in control of subtle psycho-somatic transformation.

Similar to what Peter Brook was to pursue in his intercultural theatre, travel and expedition became means of finding experiences that provided a feeling of deeper interconnectedness of self and environment. Movement exercises derived from Haitian *yanvalou* dance and singing thus blended into Grotowski's quest for what he called "objective drama" – a form that is based on craft as opposed to caprice (Slowiak and Cuesta, 2007, pp. 48–51). It was only a small step away from further exploration of the notion of ritual in Grotowski's work on the self at Pontedera. This work is primarily concerned with the levelling of energies to ever more subtle transformations to arrive at the state of organicity. Grotowski's late work with Thomas Richards mastered this creative process and resulted in Richards's work on Actions still being a part of the training in Italy today (Slowiak, 2007, p. 53).

Towards no-self: Organic movement and sacred dance

Although working from different ends of the dance/theatre spectrum, Martha Graham's dance and Jerzy Grotowski's theatre meet at the sacred centre of the body. Both of their psycho-physical explorations of Jungian archetype and myth lead to the realization that our bodily anatomy and autonomous nervous system are interconnected and mobilized through subtle movements of the spine, yogic breathing patterns or chanting using the vocal resonators. Grotowski's pioneer call for a "poor theatre" compares to Martha Graham's famous dictum that "movement never lies" (1991, p. 4). Both practitioners turn the theatrical gaze back onto the experiential body by emphasizing its inner impulses and rhythms as conveyors of felt truth. No longer a mere spectacle to watch – even though Martha Graham and Ryszard Cieślak certainly were that, too, for the mere energy their performances radiated and displayed – these theatrical bodies withdrew from representation to self-transcending realms of ritual, mysticism and embodied spirituality.

Grotowski's actor training and Martha Graham's modern dance share a concern over the sources of human expressiveness brought about by their contact with Eastern cultures. Their somewhat Primitivist quest appropriated elements from various indigenous cultures and traditions (South Asian, Native American, Caribbean and African) as it appeared motivated by a concern and search for human essence in the context of fascism and its traumatic aftermath at the end of the Second World War. Humanity then was devastated by the Holocaust and the threat of nuclear extinction of the planet as a consequence of Hiroshima and the subsequent confrontation that was the Cold War between Russia and the United States. In light of these political events, Grotowski's concern over "organicity" (Slowiak and Cuesta, 2007, pp. 7–8) sought to realign human existence at the core of nature and environmental concerns while Martha Graham's mythological works of the 1940s were very much concerned with healing a traumatized personal and national psyche (see Franko, 2012). During the phase of paratheatre, Grotowski's theatre became increasingly concerned with the synchronization of inner and outer freedom by finding oneself and thus transforming society (Slowiak and Cuesta, 2007, p. 9).

From a postmodern perspective Grotowski and Graham are oftentimes criticized for their presumably outdated assumption of a human essence at the heart of their work, and yet it seems that this quest for truthful somatic experience and expression is precisely the reason so many actors and dancers are still drawn towards their modes of training. It is interesting to compare these techniques cross-culturally as well, because they reverberate strongly with similar movement structures from non-Western dance forms which make use of singing and dancing as holistically integrated performative acts of cultural memory – precisely vehicles to communicate with one's sacred centre providing access to our inner God(dess) – and survival. Kundalini, Chi and Ashé – to be discussed in more detail later on – speak of creative energy that permeates all life on this planet. Perhaps these non-Western concepts allow for a better understanding of the essence of the transformative energy that underlies lived human and non-human existence on earth. Such cross-cultural explorations appear to critique overstated notions of cultural relativism and difference, because indeed these songs of tradition have existed in Europe as elsewhere over time. Rather it appears that Western civilization and rationalism sit uncomfortably next to their own archetypal shadow that suppresses life as its own sacred centre not to be abused and exploited. Perhaps this is based in Western guilt when confronting its own colonial past founded on the extinction of indigenous populations and beliefs, the oppression of women and, last but not least, very important truths of our own psyches at a deeper level which is yet another aspect of the political analysis we will come to later on.

Study Questions:

1. How can we compare Martha Graham's technique to Jerzy Grotowski's performer training?
2. What is the relationship between habitus, embodiment and archetype?
3. Both Graham and Grotowski subscribed to the belief that the body's memory transcends our autobiographical self and speaks its own truth. How so? Refer back to your understanding of Chapters 1 and 2.

5 Resurrecting the Dancing Chorus in the 1960s

Peter Brook's *Marat/Sade* (1964), The Living Theatre's *Antigone* (1967) and Richard Schechner's *Dionysus in 69* (1969)

In lament of the dead: Resurrecting the dancing chorus in the theatre of the 1960s

The 1960s in the United States has been described as a period of countercultural revolution by a newly emerging left-wing politics after McCarthyism, celebrating youth as a value in itself, and heralded by the 1950s rebel icons such as James Dean or Jackson Pollock, who died at their peak – sacrificial epitomes of the 1950s era of suburban affluence, media hype and mobility. Todd Gitlin in *The Sixties* summarized the appeal of the period: "You put your body on the line. Actions were believed to be the guarantees and preconditions of ideas" (1993, p. 84). Referencing the earlier avant-garde from Antonin Artaud to Surrealism, "taking up the bodies" in 1968 was hardly a new idea, yet it articulated the dissatisfaction of the beginning of the twentieth century with materialist culture and its visually driven, representational regimes of power distribution and bourgeois ideology. Following the previous discussions of Artaud, Brecht, Graham and Grotowski, the 1960s continuously imagined the moving body as the last vestige of truthful experience, connecting the alienated teenager to his or her deeper rhythms of a life worth living – a means of physical transcendence to reach beyond the trauma and anxiety of fascism, the Second World War, Cold War, nuclear threat and extinction of the human race.

Herbert Marcuse's influential *Eros and Civilization* (1998) first published in 1955 reinterpreted Freud by rephrasing the philosophy of repressed desire in a Marxist vein, and the discovery of quantum physics appealed to a public sense of energy surplus floating freely among rebelling students in the inner city streets. It is no surprise therefore that body politics took hold of a generation's imagination, and the body itself became the experimental playground of 1960s youth culture, where instant relief was found in the outlet of popular music and festival culture such as in Woodstock 1969. As Todd Gitlin recalls the communal impact of such body politics and their public display:

> I was drawn into a circle of energy, then, whose bonds were intellectual and moral, poetical and sexual at once. I must have half-imagined the chance I might be admitted – not so much to sex as such, I think, but to the mutual love and reliance and the sense of possibility which sex can stand for. Even to be in the presence of all this transpersonal libido awed me. That it should accompany intelligence and political passion seemed to prove that thought, morality, and feeling could form a whole way of life. (1993, p. 109)

Erotic transgression in the 1960s appeared to pick up on Martha Graham's call for the pelvis as the woman's sacred centre of creativity and expression asking for more than just the individual fulfilment of the Freudian pleasure principle or Jungian individuation for that matter.

The climactic, almost Dionysian, outbreaks of 1968 may therefore be read as the resurrection of the Greek dancing chorus, a ritualistic veneration of intimate psychological desires physically released to voice the dissatisfaction of the people with a society dominated by consumerist values leading into yet another war in Vietnam. Julia Kristeva's (*1941) recollection of the French student revolt furthermore suggests that we consider the impetus of 1968 as a post-Nietzschean rebellious act of re-evaluation in its denunciation of capitalist consumerism and the fascist past bearing in mind the European context (2002). The year 1968 appears to have suggested a grass-roots democratic longing towards desire-driven liberation, as in Julia Kristeva's terms an "unalterable, infinite, absolute and destructive" impulse, to seize power from the previous generation, mainly the fathers (2002, p. 26). Theatre in the 1960s thus staged the possibility of communal belonging in a celebration of a body–mind cosmological continuity existing in interdependence with the universe and natural environment. The three performances discussed in this chapter appear to resurrect the Greek dancing chorus as they devised several improvisatory exercises bypassing over-rationalization of the dramatic text and facilitate ensemble play. While Brecht, Artaud and Grotowski were direct reference points for all of them, we see how their investigation of the chorus approximates structural elements we found in Martha Graham's dance and choreography deconstructing patterns of habitual behaviour and destabilizing the social mask as part of the constitution of archetypal character work.

Furthermore, we examine in this chapter how a continued investment in archetype informs the physical exploration and interpretation of classical dramatic text focusing on the three archetypal heroes: Dionysus, Antigone and De Sade. From an archetypal perspective that they share in common, they each individually rebel against state law and oppression. Their ethical demands are thus founded on natural law, and their performance pays tribute to the experiential body as felt in ecstasy, grief and pain. As we discussed in Chapter 1, these are core-conscious emotions that characterize human existence. All three protagonists challenge their opponents in different ways and yet their common fight is against the principle of over-rationalization and the privileging of the mind as a separate, disembodied entity. Thus, Dionysus challenges Pentheus, Antigone counters Kreon and De Sade finds his rival in the perverted rationalism of the revolutionary Marat. At the same time Antigone, the Bacchae and Corday are avenging women under the rule of the Dionysian principle of the sacred feminine. Dionysus the androgynous god, half a man and half a woman, is the embodiment of eroticism, the creative life force reconciled at the sacred spot or pelvic core running up the spine where it connects to the brain. The bacchic dances symbolize the creative–erotic impulse that drives those women towards violence which avenges the social wrong and oppression symbolized by the state. They lead the chorus against a state that has become an institutionalized monster justifying a gas chamber, guillotine or war as denominator of the common good.

The three companies that we look at in this chapter were all part of the 1960s countercultural revolt, most outspoken perhaps is the Living Theatre under Judith Malina and Julian Beck. Richard Schechner and *The Performance Group* as well as Peter Brook at the time were also immersed in the raised energy levels that ignited a storm against war, fascism and oppression. In examining the dancing body and corporeality in this chapter, we see how these performances sought to define freedom and liberation in terms of community and ensemble work.

Dismantling Western maladies: Performance in the 1960s

Much has been written about the 1960s counterculture, and many of its legends continue to influence our contemporary pop culture: Jimi Hendrix, The Doors, Bob Dylan, but also Yoko Ono and John Lennon are but a few that come immediately to mind. The spirit of Woodstock and the children of flower power articulated a rebellion against the militarization and consumerism of American society, while Europe was still recovering from the devastation of the Second World War leaving Germany separated into East and West by the Berlin Wall and Poland under Russian Communist siege. To many the world indeed had become mad, and sanity was but a mere camouflage of an escapist status quo. As Foucault in his *Madness and Civilization* points out, art and madness pose an ethical question to the spectator under such political conditions. He comments: "The moment when, together, the work of art and madness are born and fulfilled is the beginning of the time when the world finds itself arraigned by that work of art and responsible before it for what it is" (Foucault, 2007, p. 272). It is therefore no accident that Peter Brook's *Marat/Sade* is perhaps the seminal twentieth-century theatre performance – saved for posterity by the 1967 film production – as Brook's direction brought together Artaudian and Brechtian principles epitomizing the Western struggle over the legacy of its own past. The lurking fascism that we already explored as the dark underbelly of Artaud's poetic writing surfaced in the dystopia of modernity as it resulted in the killing of the revolution's own children. The guillotine, concentration camp and the gulag appeared as the looming shadow of Western progress ever since the eighteenth-century Enlightenment thereby posing the question of art's responsibility in the face of so many innocent deaths.

As we have examined in the previous chapters, modernity since the seventeenth century had slowly eroded Western trust in the inner soul to let its yearning inform our feeling-toned perception of the world rather than the rational abstractions of mathematical formulas and geometric designs we follow today. René Descartes (1596–1650) and Galileo Galilei (1564–1642) are the two founding figures of rationalism and modern science; they introduced abstracted forms and figures increasingly detached from our own feeling-toned response to the world. Increasingly, the sensual body was no longer held as the proof of life as experienced by our senses, but mistrusted as deceptive and unreal (see Abram, 1996). Instead reality became increasingly located outside the body, and sense perception consequently invested in the rational-analytic examination of material objects as if those were completely detached from our inner experience. Geometry in the seventeenth century became the science of abstract form which replaced sensual reality with materialistic rationalism. This founds the epistemological shift from an inwardly felt sensual body (spirit/soul) perceived as sacred towards a scientific body (object/matter) that was profane. Hence, the history of Western civilization, industrialization, modernization and capitalism venerates the reality of body objectification although paradoxically our body is never merely an object to our own experience to recall Csordas' argument from Chapter 1.

Historically, these earlier developments in science and philosophy culminated in the French Revolution starting with the storming of the Bastille in Paris on 14 July 1789 as the first effort to liberate the people from the control of the all-powerful monarchy and clergy at the time. However, within only a few years, warring factions led to unimaginable outbursts of violent executions known as the Terror (1793–1794) burying hopes for a more liberated and just society. When Napoleon took over as First Consul in 1799, French society slowly transformed into France's First Republic, however, crowning yet another emperor to lead several wars against other European countries in the next few years. Without going further into the details of history here – which you may do in your further reading and research – the French Revolution is therefore always considered as a somewhat flawed emancipation which resulted in several later wars of liberation and ultimately led to a pervasive doubt over Enlightenment ideals as they were so often corrupted by the ones in power.

Written in 1963 by German documentary playwright Peter Weiss, *Marat/Sade* took up the tradition of German political theatre in presenting audiences with a complex historical experiment juxtaposing the years of the Terror with a time nine years after Napoleon's coup in France arguing across the murderous divide at the heart of the new state. Marat and de Sade hence function as the archetypal Janus face of violence and empowerment: while Marat as the key leader of the French Revolution sees violence for the sake of mass liberation as the last resort of the revolutionary fight, de Sade objects to any violence that is not in pursuit of individual pleasure fulfilment. Both de Sade and Marat therefore perform as advocates of violence at the heart of human existence which is conceived of as a struggle for power and domination. While the Sadist fantasy represents the individualistic morale of hedonism – such as propagated by the wealthy classes into our own contemporary capitalist system – Marat's perverted rationalization of the Terror represents the emptiness of a revolutionary promise when it turns against its own ideals. Ultimately, both positions are inhumane as they fail to acknowledge, not to mention protect, the sacredness of life. Charlotte Corday turns against Marat, yet she, too, is corrupted by de Sade's violent scheme. The play hence demonstrates the viciousness of the Western mind as solely driven by either its animalistic lusts or an unhealthy over-rationalization. Peter Weiss's play lends itself to an examination of the consequences that led Western history to betray its own ideals, pointing towards the psychological schism at the heart of the Western body–mind split. As theatre turned increasingly towards dance – as this generation of 1960s theatre makers seem to further promote – body and mind were slowly realigned.

From method to ensemble: The Theatre of Cruelty Workshop (1963)

In 1963 Peter Brook, arguably one of Britain's most acclaimed theatre directors to the present day, teamed up with the American Charles Marowitz to form an ensemble of twelve notoriously underpaid but highly motivated actors to explore what came to be known as the "Theatre of Cruelty Workshop" of the Royal Shakespeare Company, then under the guidance of Peter Hall. Although Charles Marowitz was no longer involved by the time of the actual rehearsal process for *Marat/Sade*, the workshops he and Peter Brook conducted for the Royal Shakespeare Company in 1963 appeared to set up the ensemble style acting that was to become the hallmark of this landmark production. Similar to Grotowski's approach, Marowitz was not so much discarding Stanislawski's methods as such, but started to invest personal memory associations in chance-based, ever-changing circumstances so that the logic of consequential performance was disrupted. Initially, the actor's work – not unlike that of the dancer – was primarily based on rhythm as Marowitz explains,

> Eventually rhythm, a generalized and over-used word in the theatre, got re-defined in exact, physical terms. Not only did actors experience the basic changes of rhythm – slow, fast, moderate – but the endless combinations and counterpoints that rhythms were capable of. Shortly, the same attitude the actors had taken to their objects was applied to their voices and bodies. [...] Little by little, we insinuated the idea that the voice could produce sounds other than grammatical combinations of the alphabet, and that the body, set free, could begin to enunciate a language which went beyond text, beyond psychological implication and beyond monkey-see-monkey-do facsimiles of social behaviourism. And most important of all, that these sounds and moves could communicate feelings and ideas. (1966, p. 155)

Through this work, a sense of visceral communication was discovered to create the physical language of the acting ensemble. As Marrowitz explains, contact between ensemble members was based in physical improvisation techniques:

> Contact doesn't mean staring in the eyes of your fellow actor for all you're worth. It means being so well tuned in that you can see him without looking. It means, in rare cases being linked by a group rhythm which is regulated almost physiologically – by blood circulation or heart palpitation. It is the sort of thing that exists between certain kith and kin; certain husbands and wives; certain kinds of lovers or bitter enemies. (1966, p. 159)

The main incentive of the exercises was to access physical responses from a core-conscious memory to allow for more immediate and surprising expressions than the already familiar social conventions.

Upon opening *Marat/Sade* at the Aldwych Theatre London in 1964, Peter Brook considered the importance and strength of Peter Weiss's text consisting in the evocation of "a series of impressions; little dabs, one after another, fragments of information or feeling in a sequence which stir the audience's perception" (2006 [1965], p. 5). Brook's attempt to awaken his audience via an innovative blend of Artaudian and Brechtian devices in his production of the play was in search of a new idiom. He thus sought to "make plays dense in experience" (Brook, 2006, p. 5) and create what he called a theatre of the so-called "invisible made visible" (Brook, 2008, p. 63). In *The Empty Space*, Brook's seminal collection of essays first published in 1968, the director elaborated on the importance of staging the "as if" in theatre as the possibility to explore the potential of the performer's inner self to create another world each evening. Brook explains,

> The theatre has one special characteristic. It is always possible to start again. In life this is a myth; we ourselves can never go back on anything. New leaves never turn, clocks never go back, we can never have a second chance. In the theatre the slate is wiped clean all the time. In everyday life, "if" is a fiction, in the theatre "if" is an experiment. In everyday life, "if" is an evasion, in the theatre "if" is the truth. When we are persuaded to believe in this truth, then, the theatre and life are one. (2008, p. 157)

Hence, Peter Brook does not subscribe to the idea of representation as a symbolic truth set in stone by the dramatic text, but rather a making present time and again through the live act of performance. His theatre is the Brechtian experiment combined with the sensual appeal of Artaud's heart athlete reciting poetry from the core energy articulated in both Grotowski's and Graham's physical approaches. It is for the audience to choose and make up their minds about the text, as the text itself has no truth to communicate. In the rehearsal workshops that led up to the monumental production of *Marat/Sade* that toured to New York in 1965, Brook and Marowitz attempted to break through the layers of a somewhat mechanized method acting in order to uncover degrees of madness in the performer's own body memory and core-conscious impulses and reflexes. Object associations as well as the study of madness itself helped to generate the performers' astounding physical repertoire.

Unlocking the inner self: The journey into madness

The Marquis de Sade is the central character in Weiss's play, and he proclaims that there is no meaning in revolution without the liberation of the self. Of course self-liberation had been the promise of the

Enlightenment, but how can it be achieved? As we have seen in the previous chapters of this book, the self is a complex compound of core-conscious impulses and archetypal structures formed by the proto-self and its autobiographical life experiences. While core-consciousness probably determines our most immediate and least controlled impulsive responses to the world and the environment, it is the autobiographical self as ego that most of us are primarily concerned with in terms of creating our own fictionalized sense of self-identity and who we are in the world. However, this may be a rather convincing yet false notion of control, for in fact as we have seen previously, it is not so much free will but rather pathos that drives our response to the world. For de Sade, human existence is thus defined by the transgressive experiences of the flesh in pain and ecstasy, when he proclaims,

> I learned that this is a world of bodies/ each body pulsing with a terrible power/ each body alone and racked with its own unrest/ In that loneliness/ marooned in a stone sea/ I heard lips whispering continually/ and felt all the time/ in the palms of my hands and in my skin/ touching and stroking/ Shut behind thirteen bolted doors/ my feet fettered/ I dreamed only/ of the orifices of the body/ put there/ so one may hook and twine oneself in them [...] these cells of the inner self/ are worse than the deepest stone dungeon/ and as long as they are locked/ all your revolution remains/ only a prison mutiny/ to be put down/ by corrupted fellow-prisoners (Weiss, 2006, pp. 98–99).

In many performances from Peter Brook to Pina Bausch as we will see later on, the body's bared back and naked flesh become the symbol of human vulnerability but also the boundary where the self dissolves into a larger cosmic awareness of love and givenness. When Charlotte Corday slides her hair ever so softly across de Sade's bare back accompanied by the subtle hissing of the company, it is the erotic mixture of sweet caress and violent whiplash that cuts through the audience's bones. At the same time, the chorus continues the ongoing lament of the disenfranchised impoverished masses: "Marat, we're poor, and the poor stay poor!" Exploitation of the working classes, capitalism and slavery are bound together in the legacy of the Western body–mind split of the seventeenth and eighteenth centuries. Tied to a materialist set of beliefs, body and mind were constructed as objectified entities and abstracted from a felt psycho-somatic experience of wholeness that was fundamentally exploitative of human potential and creativity. Thus, the bourgeois classes obtained power, yet the poor stayed poor.

De Sade's creed is based on mania and self-forgetting in the total experience of torture and pain afflicted upon the human body. His creed is amoral libertinism that interprets freedom as the indifference of nature towards human fate. Libertinism asserts itself in destruction and inscribes its own set of rules to obliterate the sacred givenness of life; it is the early suicidal voice of existentialism where death equals ultimate power and liberation. As in Lacan's psychoanalytic reading, one can thus argue that a forced death by torture or murder signifies the point at which the very cycles of the transformations of nature are most powerfully annihilated (1992, p. 248). Marat, on the other hand, debates ideas as the highest level of human destiny and invention. The modern self is based on the principles of action and compassion as the foundations of an emerging human rights ethics. Marat, as well, is the melancholy man who is betrayed by his own expectations as the dynamic of the liberated masses exceeds his rational control and sweeps into a bloodbath of mass violence. The frustration that results in his suffering and somatic skin disease symbolize the embodiment of the Western malady itself. His performance asks seminal questions about our human existence: Is liberation of the self even possible? And what kind of society could support and protect the self against its own destructive enemy at the core? Both mania and melancholia share, however, the belief that it is force which drives human beings in the first instance. But what is this force, if it was not for life itself given in the flesh?

Marat/Sade in New York (1965): Theatre and counterculture

The production's limited engagement in New York reverberated strongly with the emerging countercultural sentiment of many avant-garde theatre practitioners as evidenced in the edited reprint of an after-performance discussion forum with Peter Brook, Ian Richardson (Marat), Geraldine Lust, Leslie Fiedler and Gordon Rogoff edited by Richard Schechner for the *Tulane Drama Review* in 1966. While for Lust the production hit right at the "core of the human condition" (Brook et al, 1966, p. 214), it seemed to raise political issues particularly relevant to the American context of war and countercultural revolution where extreme leftist positions bordered right onto extreme right-wing rhetoric and ideology. Along the sane–insane spectrum a character such as de Sade presented the unresolved contradiction of human nature as Fiedler asserts, "Sade is sane because he has come to terms with the madness within himself: he stands outside of his own madness instead of twitching with it or sinking into catatonic immobility because of it" (Brook et al, 1966, p. 221). The encounter with one's own madness then is part of the performer's quest and archetypal exploration which seeks to overcome or liberate the locked inner selves within the body (Brook et al, 1966, p. 235). That this is a potentially dangerous quest was expressed by Ian Richardson who played Marat in Peter Brook's cast. He recalls,

> We very carefully improvised the ending. It's rather curious and frightening that when we reach that part of the play something deep down does tend to take over. We have had actual physical violence of a very serious sort breaking out: there's been real blood up there, fractured teeth, unconscious people. (Brook et al, 1966, p. 222)

While the philosophical battle is between de Sade and Marat's distinct positions, the overall conflict critiques the absolutism of ideology and its inherent terrorization of the people.

Prompted by de Sade the inmates never leave their condition as the insane according to the play-within-the-play logic. If to be insane is the nature of the human condition, there is no sane perspective to argue from as all the roles are being given by de Sade. Is de Sade a sadistic god then? The God of Nihilism? Especially, since Weiss's documentary style chooses to present actual historical speeches as a dramatic montage, by which the audience is cast as the performer's counterpart rather than the other characters on stage. And yet, Brook's assault on the audience is carefully distinguished from a mere drugging of the audience as he explains,

> You start with the fact that a vital performance – by that I mean one in which a lot of energy is engendered by stage events – is better than a deadly one. If the audience is the open vessel ready to take all this stuff in, the experience stops at that pure drug experience. What comes out of this is another possibility: the audience comes back to the play and takes from it what truly concerns it. (Brook et al, 1966, p. 231)

Ultimately, Brook's quest is very similar to Grotowski's search for organicity in that both were fundamentally interested in the performer's liberation of the self. As Peter Brook further asserts,

> The actor has to be open, not closed. If he happens to be dumb and blind he shouldn't apply for the part. Freedom alone doesn't give him the ability to exchange something with an audience. That ability comes through the actor's ability to create an object, like any other object, which exists between him and the audience; something he recognizes as absolutely true at that moment, and which the audience recognizes. (Brook et al, 1966, p. 236)

For Brook the material object does not exist as a scientific truth but is performed in the mutual encounter between the actor and his or her audience. It is based on the recognition of the other's humaneness that allows us to communicate and create a world in the making. This is the revolutionary gestus of Brook's work rooted in a phenomenology of the invisible-made-visible. It is not theatre as institutionalized pseudo-religion of entertainment, but deeply spiritual as it is based on a mutual leap of intuited faith where the "as-if" and its potential for political change become the ultimate reality of performance again and again.

Theatre of the invisible-made-visible: Peter Brook and Maurice Merlau-Ponty

Peter Brook's *The Empty Space* is a compilation of lectures he delivered at several UK universities at the time and presents us with an early reflection of Brook's theatrical quest. It is broadly divided into four chapters in which he differentiates between four different types of theatre: 1. The Deadly Theatre, 2. The Holy Theatre, 3. The Rough Theatre and 4. The Immediate Theatre. We also find in this book the often-quoted definition of theatre by which Peter Brook states, "I can take any empty space and call it a bare stage. A man walks across this empty space whilst someone else is watching him, and this is all that is needed for an act of theatre to be engaged" (2008, p. 11). As we will see, this minimal definition is derived from his critique of prevalent stage realism, which he also referred to as "deadly theatre" (Brook, 2008, pp. 11–46).

But why deadly? Peter Brook calls realist theatre deadly because it is primarily a theatre for the box-office, which uses "[r]ed curtains, spotlights, blankverse and laughter" to entertain and distract the audience from their everyday lives and problems (2008, p. 11). It is a consumerist theatre for a consumerist society.

As deadly as its aesthetic choices is also the academic theatregoer, because he does not allow for himself or herself to make new, challenging experiences, but rather seeks a confirmation of his intellectual understanding of the given play text (2008, p. 13). Peter Brook explains,

> If we talk of deadly, let us note that the difference between life and death, so crystal clear in man, is somewhat veiled in other fields. [...] how an idea, an attitude or a form can pass from the lively to the moribund. [...] all the printed word can tell us is what was written on paper, not how it was once brought to life. [...] the best dramatists explain themselves the least. [...] They recognize that the only way to find the true path to speaking of a word is through the process that parallels the original creative one. (2008, pp. 13–15)

This quote challenges us to find our own new meaning in each dramatic text we perform. Peter Brook was an ardent lover of Shakespeare, and we owe to this creative genius some of the most wonderful Shakespeare productions, for example his *Lear* (1962) and *Midsummer Night's Dream* (1970). But what then can we do to avoid the deadly and still approach of the performance of a classic dramatic text?

Not unlike Martha Graham and Jerzy Grotowski, Peter Brook suggests that each generation of theatre artists will have to find their own style and interpretation of the classic repertoire engaging the archetypal layer to create innovative stage imagery. He suggests that "great theatre is not a fashion house" (2008, p. 19) and that we therefore need to avoid incompetence (2008, p. 35) and repetition (2008, p. 44) by not using old formulae and methods but rather find our own modes of expression. Finally, he compares the deadly theatre to the deadly bore – someone who is likewise amusing perhaps but not to be taken seriously. Because that is what Peter Brook ultimately wants: for us to take theatre seriously so that it becomes a necessity in our lives. And this is what Peter Brook then calls "The Holy Theatre" (2008, p. 63). Brook defines holy theatre by saying rather mysteriously that it is the "invisible-made-visible" – as if that would clarify anything! Yet, can you perhaps think of what this may mean in light of this book's earlier discussion of the Artaudian double, Martha Graham's inner landscape or Jerzy Grotowski's state of grace, for example? Think also about this suggestion by philosopher Giorgio Agamben (*1942), when he talks about the significance of play in a secular world saying: "This means that play frees and distracts humanity from the sphere of the sacred, without simply abolishing it. The use to which the sacred is returned is a special one that does not coincide with utilitarian consumption" (2007, p. 76). Similarly, Peter Brook suggests that we should create images in the theatre that are derived from a felt inner impulse bypassing the consumerist user value of performance. Such images and gestures carry a feeling-charged memory that is based in our physical response which is partly based in our individual experience, but they also exceed our experience as they are expressive of an ongoing embodied life force that connects one generation to the next.

Brook gives an example of this, when he relates the holy theatre to our experience of music, but he also refers to Samuel Beckett as a playwright and Merce Cunningham, the choreographer, who we will look at in the next chapter. In that respect, holy theatre is drawn to ritual and dance. Peter Brook, similar to Artaud, therefore wants his theatre to be infectious and sacred in that sense, although relevant for audiences in contemporary society. Brook shares Artaud's belief in the power of affective images, when he says,

> What he [Artaud] wanted in his search for holiness was absolute: he wanted a theatre that would be a hallowed place; he wanted that theatre served by a band of dedicated actors and directors who would create out of their own natures an unending succession of violent stage images, bringing about such powerful immediate explosions of human matter that no one would ever again revert to a theatre of anecdote and talk. (2008, pp. 59–60)

However, Brook was also sceptical of Artaud's fascist tendencies and asked several critical questions one should also bear in mind, when working from and with core energetic impulses:

- Is Artaud's vision creative–therapeutic?
- Or rather fascist–destructive?
- Or is it a denial of the mind?

These questions demonstrate how difficult it is to create a notion of holiness in contemporary theatre performance. Peter Brook firmly believed in the importance of the audience as well as in the function of theatre as communication. His definition of holy theatre therefore summarizes that what we ultimately need to strive for is not only holy art, which makes the invisible essence of organic life visible, but also create the necessary conditions to allow for such self-transformative experience. He says, "In any event, to comprehend the visibility of the invisible is a life's work. Holy art is an aid to this, and so we arrive at a definition of holy theatre. A holy theatre not only presents the invisible but also offers conditions that make its perception possible" (2008, p. 63).

If holy theatre is at the opposite extreme of deadly theatre, then there are two more forms of theatre Peter Brook is interested in. One of which is the so-called "rough theatre" (2008, p. 76). Rough theatre refers to all the popular theatre forms that we find in carnival, satire, games, etc. Peter Brook cherishes this theatre, because he considers it "anti-authoritarian, anti-traditional, anti-pomp, anti-pretence" (2008, p. 76). Rough theatre is the theatre of and by the people, and we find examples of that in Shakespeare's fools, or Alfred Jarry's *Ubu Roi* (1896). He also gives the example of Brecht's use of gestus and alienation as well as 1960s Happenings. Both forms, he argues, make us look again, see something as if for the first time so we can recognize a different perspective and outlook on life (2008, p. 81).

The "immediate theatre", lastly, is the kind of theatre that emerges in the instant. Peter Brook was famous for using a workshop format for rehearsal where actors would be free to improvise and find their own forms of expression. This is a style that considers practicality as important, and it emphasizes the process of creation. Peter Brook says that "there are no formulae, there are no methods" and "no permanence", whereby he means that each expression needs to emerge from ensemble work. The work of the group, which he as the director, then, orchestrates, is important. He describes his work with actors as similar to gardening: "An actor, like any artist, is like a garden and it is no help to pull out the weeds just once, for all time. The weeds always grow, this is quite natural, and they must be cleaned away, which is natural and necessary too" (2008, p. 128). Immediacy then is essential, if we want to create the conditions for holy theatre to emerge. It means that we need to make the past our contemporary, and in order to do so we need to find our own meaning in every text that we perform. Peter Brook refers to this process as re-presentation – meaning to present again – and in a new and exciting way thereby creating an image that makes us see reality for the first time each instance:

> [A] representation denies time. It abolishes that difference between yesterday and today. It takes yesterday's action and makes it live again every one of its aspects – including its immediacy. In other words, a representation is what it claims to be – a making present. We can see how this is the renewal of the life that repetition denies and it applies as much to rehearsal as to performance. (2008, p. 155)

If we create this kind of theatre, then we are a step removed from our habitual concepts of what reality is and should look like. Indeed, we are cherishing life's creativity as holy and intact.

Maurice Merleau-Ponty: Experiencing the (In)Visible

As a key thinker of phenomenology, Maurice Merleau-Ponty's philosophy shares an interest in dismantling the invisible as a source of organic life that we can fruitfully discuss alongside the examples discussed so far. According to Merleau-Ponty, perception is our inner sense – not unlike Jung's concept of the collective unconscious – that allows us to ascribe meaning to the world as we can see, hear, touch and smell it. Merleau-Ponty stresses that reality is not merely a fact but needs to be carefully described at each instance, as our experiences are mostly formed by our imaginary and dreams (2004, p. xi). Phenomenology is thus intricately bound up with the analysis of our inner world and dreams. As Merleau-Ponty claims, "In dreaming as in myth we learn where the phenomenon is to be found, by feeling that towards which our desire goes out, what our heart dreads, on what our life depends (Merleau-Ponty, 2004, p. 333). In the daily abundance of our experiences and perceptions, he thus believed that each meaning we ascribe is only one of further possibilities (Merleau-Ponty 2004, p. 40).

However, rather unlike Jung, Merleau-Ponty asserts that we have knowledge only of our own present which as such enables us to perceive of the ideas of ego, truth and objectivity (Merleau-Ponty, 2004, p. 51). Compared to Bergson's belief in intuition as our felt core-conscious response, Merleau-Ponty's vision appears much more analytical as well, since he emphasizes our capacity to reveal and thus explain "the prescientific life of consciousness" (Merleau-Ponty, 2004, p. 68). According to Merleau-Ponty, the body is hence primarily perceived as a "temporal structure" of successive instances in time. Each moment bears the trace of the previous one and builds further events from there (Merleau-Ponty, 2004, p. 162). Merleau-Ponty points out, "I am not in space and time, nor do I conceive space and time; I belong to them, my body combines with them and includes them" (2004, p. 162). Part one of *Phenomenology of Perception* thus addresses the problem of "The Body" more specifically as "the vehicle of being in the world [...] intervolved in a definite environment" (Merleau-Ponty, 2004, pp. 94–95). As such the body is seen as our "medium for having a world" by positing biological, figurative and cultural meanings, as well as constituting its motor habits (Merleau-Ponty, 2004, p. 169). Merleau-Ponty defines "body" as follows:

> Body experience forces us to acknowledge an imposition of meaning which is not the work of a universal constituting consciousness, a meaning which clings to certain contents. My body is that meaningful core which behaves like a general function, and which nevertheless exists, and is susceptible to disease. In it we learn to know that union of essence and existence which we shall find again in perception generally, and which we shall then have to describe more fully. (2004, p. 170)

Merleau-Ponty compares the body to an artwork in the sense that pictures or music are also understood as the sum of their component parts such as sounds, colours and instruments (2004, p. 174). The only way of experiencing our body is therefore by "living it", thinking about the body will not present us with any knowledge of what the body is (Merleau-Ponty, 2004, p. 231).

Hence, the body helps us to orient our projects as a means of existing in the world. As humans we need "to build into the geographical setting a behavioural one, a system of meanings outwardly expressive of the subject's internal activity" (Merleau-Ponty, 2004, p. 129). Merleau-Ponty therefore defines consciousness as the power which gives meaning to experience and runs parallel to the body, as self-awareness must be either all-inclusive or not existing at all

(Merleau-Ponty, 2004, pp. 139–142). Movement is therefore crucial for us to understand ourselves, as he concludes,

> Motility, then, is not, as it were, a handmaid of consciousness, transporting the body to that point in space of which we have formed a representation beforehand. In order that we may be able to move our body towards an object, the object must first exist for it, our body must not belong to the realm of the "in-itself". [...] We must therefore avoid saying that our body is in space, or in time. It inhabits space and time. (2004, p. 142)

While taking a scientific approach, Merleau-Ponty also critiques intellectualism and science for their "commonplace utterances" and institutionalized meanings, when he suggests that we rather focus on the "ready-made meanings" we already possess as our own subjective awareness of the world (2004, p. 213). He argues that by refocusing our attention on the gestural component of words as well as their sounding qualities we may experience what he refers to as their "emotional essence" (2004, p. 217). This is an interesting turning point, as it observes the potential for aesthetic reimagining (Merleau-Ponty, 2004, pp. 212–213). The same applies, so he argues, when it comes to gesture: "It is not enough for two conscious subjects to have the same organs and nervous system for the same emotions to produce in both the same signs. What is important is how they use their bodies, the simultaneous patterning of body and world in emotion" (2004, p. 220). Instead of buying into naturalistic realism, Merleau-Ponty thus subscribes to a reinstatement of a mythic space of "affective entities" which precede our perception and determine our existence. Similar to Artaud he compares the feeling to the rhythm patterns of the tides or the systole/diastole of our pulsing heart beats as source of organic life (2004, pp. 332–333).

In his later work *The Visible and the Invisible* (1968) Merleau-Ponty returns to the distrust in science as it is rather our experience that brings meaning into the world which ultimately transcends conventions of literalism and total explication. Human experience calls for language, yet maintains a structural openness of signification that cannot be referred back, although the underlying energetic essence of the ever-present life force may be revealed. Merleau-Ponty explains, "In the midst of the sensuous experience there is an intuition of an essence, a sense, a signification. The sensible is the place where the invisible is captured in the visible" (1968, p. xli). Whereas the visible appears as "the sensible thing [which] is exterior to the being of the subject" (Merleau-Ponty, 1968, p. xlvii), the invisible as "the very manner of the visible" marks out the space between things as their "fields of possible variation in the same thing and in the same world" (Merleau-Ponty, 1968, pp. l–li). Paradoxically, the invisible makes visibility possible as without it there would be no recognition whatsoever. Merleau-Ponty describes this process:

> With the first vision, the first contact, the first pleasure, there is initiation, that is, not the positing of a content, but the opening of a dimension that can never again be closed, the establishment of a level in terms of which every other experience will henceforth be situated. The idea is this level, this dimension. It is therefore not a de facto invisible, like an object hidden behind another, and not an absolute invisible, that would have nothing to do with the visible. Rather it is the invisible of this world, that which inhabits this world, sustains it, and renders it visible, its own and interior possibility, the Being of this being. (1968, p. 151)

In James Hillman's psychoanalytic terms, the invisible could thus be described as the soul or Jungian archetype underlying our capacity to perceive and experience the world as intensely alive (see Moore, 1989).

Our imaginary thus produces an abundance of inner and outer images which Merleau-Ponty refers to as "the 'baroque' proliferation of generating axes for visibility in the duplicity of the real" (Merleau-Ponty, 1968, p. liii). What Merleau-Ponty describes as "flesh" is our inwardly felt subjective experience of response – the body as a sensing organism to enable our seeing, touching, hearing and smelling as originary moments of subjective corporeity and meaning enlivened by emotional context (1968, p. liv). Similar to Damasio earlier on in the book, Merleau-Ponty also chooses the theatre as a metaphor for perception whereby our eyes function as the "curtains" opened onto a world where our body is the "stage director" of our lives:

> [M]y body as stage director of my perception has shattered the illusion of a coinciding of my perception with the things themselves. Between them and me there are henceforth hidden powers, that

> whole vegetation of possible phantasms which it holds in check only in the fragile act of the look. No doubt, it is not entirely my body that perceives: I know only that it can prevent me from perceiving, that I cannot perceive without its permission. (1968, pp. 8–9)

Hence, Merleau-Ponty concludes that experience is more trustworthy than language which we learn how to use, yet at the same time it does not guarantee the reality of the meaning it purports (1968, p. 12). Ultimately, language then is also enigmatic rather than revealing, as it becomes "itself a world [...] since it speaks of being and of the world and therefore redoubles their enigma instead of dissipating it" (1968, p. 96). Yet, despite Merleau-Ponty's apparent mistrust in language, he also postulates a faith in the face-to-face exchange of words as in a personal conversation, or, indeed, in the theatre (Merleau-Ponty, 1968, p. 13).

At the same time, the invisible discloses meaning from us all the time, just as much as it makes meaning possible (Merleau-Ponty, 1968, p. 14). According to Merleau-Ponty, experience is thus solipsistic ("I live my perception from within, and, from within, it has an incomparable power of ontogenesis" 1968, p. 58; "I will never live any but my own life and the others will never be but other myselves" 1968, p. 71), and yet we are in constant relationship with the world as it is revealed to our understanding. The visible is hence the realm of the present instance, our power for contemplation that fixes time and place. Although we can only ever be sure of the now of visibility, there is also a haunting trace of the invisible, that instant past as well as future which Merleau-Ponty refers to as the "inextricable problem of the intuition of essences" (1968, p. 114). Therefore one can think of oneself as being here and now as much as everywhere:

> For the visible present is not in time and space, nor, of course, outside of them: there is nothing before it, after it, about it, that could compete with its visibility. And yet it is not alone, it is not everything. To put it precisely, it stops up my view, that is, time and space extend beyond the visible present, and at the same time they are behind it, in depth, in hiding. The visible can thus fill me and occupy me only because I who see it do not see it from the depths of nothingness, but from the midst of itself; I the seer am also visible. What makes the weight, the thickness, the flesh of each color, of each sound, of each tactile texture, of the present, and of the world is the fact that he who

> grasps them feels himself emerge from them by a sort of coiling up or redoubling, fundamentally homogenous with them; he feels that he is the sensible itself coming to itself and that in return the sensible is in his eyes as it were his double or an extension of his own flesh (1968, p. 114).

These lines imply a certain kind of mysticism of beyond the self, an expansive experience which transcends the ego perspective as it becomes aware of its felt affective core. Phenomenology thus points to the techniques employed by the dancers and theatre makers discussed thus far as they explored movement and its potential for creating a responsive, pre-conceptual engagement with life and experience. Their choreography emerges from the invisible yet organic source of life that pulses through the different energy centres of our anatomic body. Without those, no thinking would be possible. While theatre before the phenomenological turn had overemphasized its reliance on words and their rational meaning, dance structures emerge in actor training as a corrective rebalancing of perception and self-discovery. The body appears as the central mediator aligning invisible forces with visible expression at the heart of theatrical communication.

The Living Theatre's *Antigone*

Judith Malina's work on Antigone started with a fascination she felt for Brecht's theatre, in particular his 1948 *Antigone* which had served Helene Weigel as an earlier character exploration to prepare her for *Mother Courage* which we already discussed. As Malina recalls in her preface to the published translation of the play, it was mostly her interest in Brecht's politics of embodiment that started her exploration. Dramatic text had to be questioned by the actions and gestus of the performers and words had to be filled with sounding poetic meaning as was particularly pronounced in Hölderlin's German adaptation of Sophocles' original that Brecht had used. As we have seen with Graham and Grotowski before, the play text here serves but as a mere trace of the felt experience it was meant to convey at the time to question how it can translate into the present moment. The character exists only partially on the page. Rather the scenic arrangement – or choreography – enlivens the relationship between the performers as much as their body work developed from physical exercises and improvisations. Malina translated the text in prison – one of several detainments the Living Theatre underwent during the 1960s by state police – as part of their ongoing struggle for a pacifist world. Their company was perhaps the most outspokenly political as their theatre productions were the ones which most directly verged on immediate political protest. As Malina recalls of those days:

> It was a time of growing hopefulness that led to the enormous energy of 1968, a time of rising belief in the possibility of creating the world in which we all want to live, a time of optimism and vigorous resistance to the authoritarian aspects of the social structure which the violent past has left us as its legacy. (1990, p. v)

Equipped with her reading of Brecht and Artaud, Malina began her character work by interrogating the meaning of Antigone as a heroine of the non-violent Anarchist Revolution of that time (Malina, 1990, pp. vi–vii). Performed in more than sixteen countries from 1966 into the 1980s the Living Theatre's *Antigone* played homage to the liberation struggle that defeated those who still believed in war as an effective means of politics, whether in Ireland, Franco's Spain or Poland and Prague (Malina, 1990, p. vii).

When rehearsals for *Antigone* started in 1966, the performance became a "true celebration of civil disobedience" for everyone involved (Biner, 1972, p. 145). The Living Theatre followed Brecht in that for them, too, this plot was no longer driven by fate but larger economic forces determining world politics in the background. More than twenty performers were on stage at all times; they wore street clothes and embodied the people of Thebes throughout, while the audience was cast as Argos (Biner, 1972, p. 149).

Similar to Artaud's double then, the Living Theatre's heroine Antigone performed by Judith Malina bridged the world between the living and the dead. In times of war, the Living Theatre's set-up seemed to suggest that the dead summon the living to interrogate the meaning of life for those who survive. As Jan Kott suggests,

> In the tragic world the dead return. The tragic hero is alone among people, perhaps because he lives, like Antigone, in the world of

> the dead. In the world of those who have been murdered, or whom he has murdered himself. The dead demand, first, to be buried, but later they demand redress (1970, p. x).

Less significant than the gods' command in the Sophoclean original, the Living Theatre asks the audience to position themselves in the face of the atrocity and monstrousness of the war. Malina carefully choreographed each movement for her performance of Antigone, as well as parts for the chorus. Movement became the key element for expressing the power dynamic between characters as they not always moved on their own will, but were literally dragged around or placed in a tableau constellation by Kreon (Julian Beck). More importantly, the scenic arrangement and choreography assured that the group was facing the individual as was already characteristic of Brecht's work on gestus in the original Modellbuch Malina had studied. Moreover, the company referred performers to the study of painting and sculpture, an analysis of the significant amount of mysticism in the play text, and images of Greek vases and Egyptian burial rites to create physical imagery and visceral effects (Biner, 1972, pp. 154–155). Imitative and religious sounds were also used to create an affective atmosphere throughout (Biner, 1972, p. 149).

In the 1980 Italian TV documentation of the Living Theatre's *Antigone*, we can see how the performance began in silence. One by one, each performer entered the stage, calm and contained in their jeans and jumpers to stand still and establish eye contact with the audience. Although performed on a conventional proscenium stage, the group did not use any props or scenography throughout. Their bodies were their only means of expression. Contact with the audience was further enhanced by steps that led down into the auditorium and was frequently used by members of the chorus, but also by Kreon (Julian Beck). After several minutes of initial silence, the performers begin to create a soundscape evoking sirens and vultures screeching. Some performers kneel down on the floor and cover their heads with their arms. This continues for several minutes before Antigone (Judith Malina) and Ismene appear on stage. Kreon leads a screaming performer towards centre stage, where he is symbolically dismembered and killed – holding the place for the dead body of Polyneikes, but also representing the many young men dead and dying in Vietnam at that time.

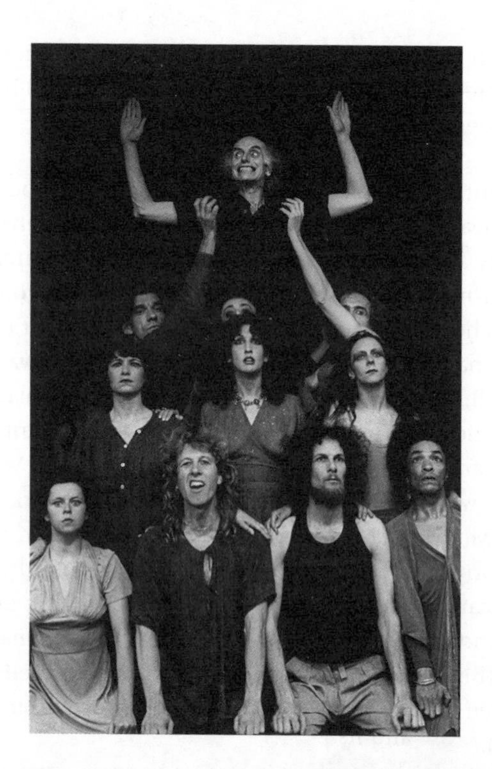

Living Theatre's *Antigone* © Bernd Uhlig.

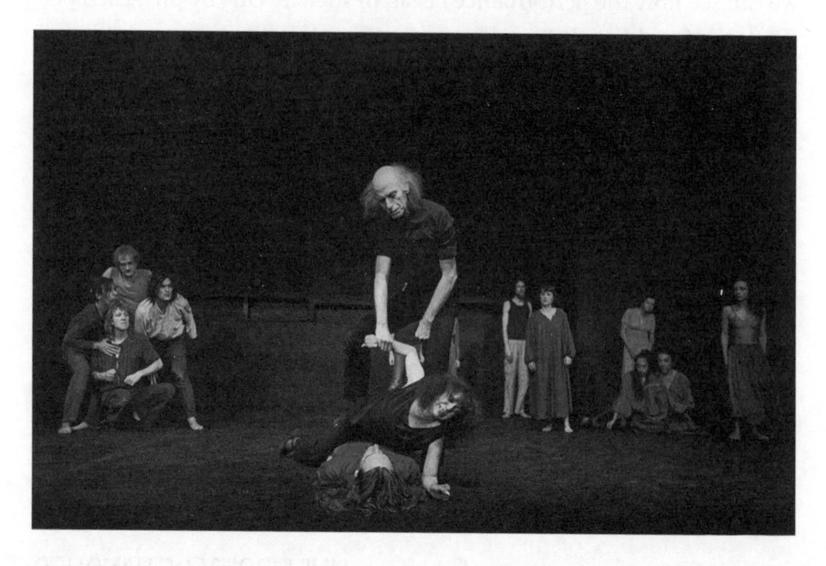

Living Theatre's *Antigone* © Bernd Uhlig.

Throughout the performance Malina returns to her characteristic gestus for the role: she gathers dust with both hands as her signature movement commenting on each scene. As Biner described in detail:

> Each gesture of depositing is accompanied by a mournful intake of breath ("haaa ..."), because the body makes contact with dead matter, followed by an eased exhalation ("heee ..."), because the life of the body communicates itself to the dead matter. Antigone's gesture is a representation of Polyneikes' resurrection in the form of a revolutionary impulse: She gives "life" to Polyneikes by rebelling, as she gives "life" to the dust she deposits in her mouth. (1972, p. 156)

Polyneikes's body remains lifeless on stage throughout as a constant reminder of the presence of death on stage. As Julian Beck explained,

> In Antigone, the constant presence on stage of the body of Ployneices acts as a magnetic pole which governs not only the play's action, but the spectator's concentration. He is the locus, the factual guilt. Until we embrace him and incorporate him into our lives we can never eradicate the doom that his death dictates to all of us. The unburied corpse and its power embody sacrificial presence. (Phelps, 1967, p. 129)

Three times during the performance the actors descend into the auditorium: first, to mime the battle in which Eteocles and Polyneikes die, second, for the famous chorus on the monstrosity of mankind, and third, when Megaros's death signifies the ongoing war in Theban society (Biner, 1972, p. 150). Although the audience in the TV production remained awkwardly calm and uncomfortable perhaps, the staging was clearly an appeal for them to get out of their comfort zone and change their lives. The dances of Bacchus performed throughout the latter half of the play with singing, clapping, stomping and hissing were a pertinent reminder that the individual's quest for freedom could not be forever subdued.

Workshop exercises

Through kinetic work, the Living Theatre's performers became Artaudian doubles of the dead among the living, heart athletes who operated in passionate time. How did they get into that stage of ecstatic performance? What exercises did they explore? While the Greeks had already referred to this heightened awareness as the state they called "mania" (see Dodds, 1951), the Living Theatre, just as those companies we considered before, attempted to find such luminosity for the performer in the contemporary world. As Julian Beck explained their approach:

> Our work is kinetic, and has to be seen – we ourselves have to see it in all its stages. We want to use the body in such a way that it contains the actor's sacrificial presence, to use kinaesthetics in the poetic theatre in such a way that the medium materializes. (Malina, quoted in: Phelps, 1967, p. 126)

If the madness of Artaud was conceived as a state of disassociation with reality, then how could such assumed schizophrenia free the performer's self from preoccupation with the ego, for example? One strategy, we can observe in the Living Theatre's *Antigone*, is to have groups of ensemble stage tableaux or act in pairs. The emotion they convey is thereby no longer individual, but determined by the group constellation and the social power dynamic at play. Instances of such tableaux in the production are the one where they stage the hear nothing, see nothing, say nothing monkeys – or when Malina and, later on, Beck lie down on the dead body in a gesture of reconciliation with the dead seeking to overcome guilt and/or redeem the human fault of war crimes, past and ongoing.

In line with the generational quest for a counterculture, the Living Theatre sought to increase the so-called "conscious awareness" (Phelps, 1967, p. 128) overcoming concerns for the ego and individualism by engaging with Eastern practices of meditation but also forms of mysticism based in the Jewish kabbala. Similar to Grotowski's methods this was primarily a quest for a new physical vocabulary that transgressed the hold of the social mask to access an organic, energetic life source. As Julian Beck described this process in their work on Brechtian alienation:

> With Antigone we have found voices for the words, and movements for the body, that differ from voice and movement as practiced in most civilized theatre. If we want to change the world physically, culturally, economically, socially, psychologically or even poetically, everything has to change. (in: Phelps, 1967, p. 128)

Again, as we have seen in Brook's ensemble work as well, the effort was to transform the individual in order to change society on a larger scale as one of the major political impetuses after the Second World War. Work on the body that verged on choreography and improvised modes of moving and dancing were crucial to achieve this energetic shift that changed theatre towards dance in the second half of the twentieth century. Joseph Chaikin who started out with the Living Theatre in the 1950s was to pursue his own work in collective ensemble theatre around the same time. His seminal book on the period is called *The Presence of the Actor* (1972) in which he talks about *The Serpent* (1968) and several other important performances of his company. Yet another influence, however, came via the exploration of a different space for performance. Increasingly theatre was no longer performed on the proscenium stage, but sought sites and environments to enhance the physical impact of the companies' body work. This is studied in the next section as we explore Richard Schechner's environmental theatre.

The Performance Group: *Dionysus in 69*

In January 1968, a couple of months after Richard Schechner and a group of fellow actors founded The Performance Group, rehearsal for *Dionysus in 69* started in a small garage on Wooster Street, New York City. About twenty young actors signed up for the initial workshops which started with an exercise of scrubbing floors to slowly transform the garage into an environmental theatre space. Environmental theatre appeared as a buzzword of the 1960s counterculture, where performance art and happenings as well as postmodern dance – discussed in the next chapter – took performance outside the institutional theatre buildings and into the streets to affect, alter and change the political sphere and public discourse.

In his *Environmental Theatre* (1994), first published 1973, Richard Schechner outlines the triangular relationship between (a) the environment, (b) the text and (c) the action. Here we can clearly see the influence of Grotowski's approach. Physical exercises focused on the visceral exploration of the space by blindfolding performers to let them focus on touch and contact as well as introduced a set of warm-up routines consisting of head rolls, backbends, runs, leaps and shoulder stands leading into associative exercises to stimulate mental processes based in physicality. The study of Greek theatre and tragedy in particular lends itself to the conceptualization of environmental theatre as it suggested an early example of a theatre that had politically impacted on the society of its time. Schechner's troupe attempted an alignment of performance and everyday life merging the two experiences of time and space as continuous rather than separate. During the rehearsal time, the text evolved as the environment was built (1994, p. 36). It was also important that rehearsal took place in the same space as the final performance so that the towers and platforms of the set directly emerged from the physical exercises and improvisations in the space.

Similarly, the audience was conceived as an active participant in the performance and integral part of the environmental structure (1994, p. 24). As Schechner commented, the best place to sit depended on what the audience wanted, which could be "involvement, distance, a place near the center of the holocaust, or somewhere long and dark and quiet enough to doze" (1970, n.p.) The central aspect of audience participation was thus to allow for physical contact and energetic transmission to create a kinaesthetic space of involvement (1994, p. 2). Schechner carefully sequenced the arrival, mixing and regrouping of audience members as to ensure that they would undergo their own transformative journey alongside the performers' actions (1994, p. 24). Space and time were carefully choreographed with audience and performers moving around each other throughout the evening's performance up to a point where everybody was dancing as part of the bacchic ritual.

One of the outstanding scenes at the beginning was the birth ritual as Schechner adapted it from the Asmats of New Guinea. In this ritual, women would intone and sing prayers to facilitate the birthing process as they consistently move in a danced pelvic contraction. Adapted for the performance, Schechner had the female performers recite the birth of Dionysus alias actor Finley in the play as follows:

> So his mother bore him once in labor bitter there is no towering man who mocked your mysteries and when the weaving fates fulfilled the time, the bull-horned god was born of what was the name of the child you bore that man? Good evening, sir, may I take you to your seat? (1970, n.p.)

As the quote indicates, the audience was explicitly welcomed into the space to interrupt the convention of realism in a Brechtian mode of alienation. Initially all performers emerge through the birth channel, and the ritual thus marks the transformation of the actor as a creative initiation whereby the undressing and nakedness of the performer's body was intended as a "sacred and surgical preparation" (1970, n.p.). The "fetal meditation" as Schechner called the specific squatting position that the performers would take thus became a physical memory of one's birth as much as a purification of the mind to focus on the act of performance (1970, n.p.).

Likewise, the floor mats assumed the function of a sacred place to facilitate the rituals of birth and death as sacred acts. As Schechner describes this process as part of shedding the performer's social mask:

> Our first experience with nakedness was in a workshop in February 1968 [...] before Dionysus opened, we rehearsed the ecstasy dance naked. We started to sense to what degree clothes were a social mask and how that mask could be worn even while naked. [...] we probed the relationship between nakedness and psychic vulnerability, eroticism, functional nudity, and private communication. (1970, n.p.)

Another important element was the exploration of sound to create the acoustic component of the environment as a vehicle for ecstatic transformation of the space. Schechner recalls,

> The ecstasy originated in experiments with music and movement, the relationships between the two, and probes into our own feelings. [...] From this early work we gained a sense of sonic environment, or "articulating space" through sound. We began to feel music as an extension of our bodies and to recognize sound as something to give and take. (1970, n.p.)

Environmental theatre was thus fundamentally an exploration of communal energy as a vehicle for revolutionary transformation. Dionysus represented an archetypal undercurrent that took hold of the entire group, not only the individual performer. As Schechner describes,

> It is this connection we celebrate in the ecstasy dance. It is in honor of Dionysus, but the Dionysus who is of The Performance Group.

> This God is creation, and his terror and beauty extensions of our own possibilities. No abstract deity handed down through literature, Dionysus in the garage is the energy of all focused through one. (1970, n.p.)

This point was further emphasized by the adopted multi-casting strategy, whereby different performers were cast in different roles throughout the run of *Dionysus in 69*. Each member of the group would be exposed to the different energetic impulses and movement qualities a specific role afforded. If you consider the digitally remastered film available on NYU's digital video library online, you can consider the extent to which energy exchange and audience/performer proximity were crucial elements for the environmental set-up of the production.

The tragic confrontation of Pentheus and Dionysus was played out as the confrontation of the American government with the protesting student revolt. *Dionysus in 69* thus resurrected the dancing chorus as a reminder of the cathartic–therapeutic powers of performance as a ritualistic remedy for social ills – as Schechner elaborated in *Between Theater & Anthropology* (1985) based on Victor Turner's study of ritual and social drama later on. Surrounded by the pathos of the Vietnam War and civil rights struggle, environmental theatre aimed at a catharsis that spilt out of the theatre and into the streets. As demanded by Sam alias the Messenger in the script that resulted from The Performance Group's rehearsal process:

> Yes, it's a death struggle. Dionysus versus Pentheus. The organism versus the law. I'm a messenger. But even if I stick to the text, it won't change a thing. I could tell you what I saw outside this garage. [...] Then Dionysus and Pentheus will rise from the pit, we'll get on with the action, and you can have a kind of mute catharsis. [...] Look, if Dionysus could lead you into the promised land, Dionysus or someone else could lead you right out again. Dig? Most of us have a pretty cheap fantasy of self-liberation. So before I open the pit door and set your catharsis in motion, consider this. It's harder to be a man than to be god. And tragedy leaves behind no morals it consumes them. So don't understand us too quickly. Dig? (1970, n.p.)

As with the previous examples, the point is to transform the self as the basis for a transformation of society. The performance consequently ended with the death ritual mirroring the adapted New Guinean ritual from the beginning. Blood-smeared, the performers descend into the abyss of the human impulse to kill and destroy. However, by the end of the performance, they emerge from the disaster with a new perspective. As Finley wipes the blood from his hands and puts on a presidential blue suit in a mock pre-election campaign, group members lift him up on their shoulders and come out of the garage into the New York City streets proclaiming,

> I am William Finley, a god by any other name. A god that smokes seven brands of cigarettes, a god that eats food, men, and women. A god with a Social Security number. But an unemployed god. Dionysus, son of William and Dorothy, and still not recognized as a true god by everyone in this garage. (1970, n.p.)

Performances during the 1960s resurrected the dancing chorus as a model of ensemble play that was influenced by the readings of Artaud and Grotowski and further enriched by the anthropological writings of Victor Turner (1920–1983) on ritual and social drama. Turner's definition of "communitas" describes a spontaneous, immediate and concrete gathering that brings people together around an empty centre – the mark of life – to fully interact. Unlike social structure, "communitas" references human potential on a metaphorical level expressed in art and religion (Turner, 1969). Fundamentally, "communitas" thus describes human interaction on the level of pure consciousness, which expresses our creative potential to grow as human beings. Furthermore, Turner's model conceives of communitas and social structure as dialectical processes of societal change and renewal, whereby communitas can turn into fascistic despotism if not carefully guarded. Turner's model thus posits communitas at the heart of human socialization. The discussed examples of 1960s performances express in many ways the grassroots driven longing for self-liberation that took hold of an entire generation worldwide. By resurrecting the dancing chorus in the theatre of the 1960s, performers channelled this political energy into creative work that was to transform our understanding of dance and theatre thereafter.

Study Questions:

1. Focus on the chapter "The Holy Theatre" from Peter Brook's *The Empty Space* (1968). What are some of the aesthetic elements characteristic of "holy theatre"? Is there a relationship to Artaud's notion of "affective athleticism" discussed before?
2. Peter Weiss's *Marat/Sade* presents a curious blend of Brechtian politics and Artaudian devices – choose any particular scene of the play to analyse and investigate that unlikely pairing.
3. Does Judith Malina's performance of gestus in *Antigone* provide us with an instance of Merleau-Ponty's "invisible made visible"? If yes, how so? Are there other examples discussed in this chapter you can think of?
4. What is the relationship between space and performer in Richard Schechner's concept of Environmental Theatre?
5. Explore the notion of "visceral space sense" and the workshop exercises in the chapter on "The Performer" in Richard Schechner's *Environmental Theatre* – to what extent does this spatial approach allow for a phenomenological exploration?
6. What is the relationship between theatre, ritual and dance in the theatre of the 1960s? Discuss.

6 Dance and the 1960s Counterculture

Merce Cunningham, Anne Halprin and Postmodern Dance

Mind-time in Merce Cunningham's *Walkaround Time* 1968

Compared to the theatre revolutionaries we discussed in the previous chapter, Merce Cunningham appears less of a flower power child, and yet the revolution he staged was not any less revolutionary for how people started to look at dance before and after his work. A dancer with Martha Graham in his early days, Merce Cunningham was known for his ethereal jumps – legs that took him off into the air as if gravity was not an obstacle to overcome. Merce Cunningham embodied movement incarnate as he explored the body's axes and rotations to discover what they could do that had not been done before. Dissatisfied with the psychological drama and archetypes explored in dance and theatre before him, his questions delved even deeper into the origins of life asking: what is it exactly that makes us move in the world? Do we really need to invent these stories and myths or would it be enough to just dance as a somewhat self-effacing political act to put the dancer in an immediate sphere of self-accomplishment whereby he or she simply excelled at dancing – nothing more? As Cunningham suggests,

> What the dancer does is the most realistic of all possible things, and to pretend that a man standing on a hill could be doing everything except just standing is simply divorce – divorce from life, from the sun coming up and going down, from clouds in front of the sun, from the rain that comes from the clouds and sends you into the drugstore for a cup of coffee, from each thing that succeeds each thing. Dance is a visible action of life. (Harris, 1997, p. 67)

To Peter Brook, after all, Cunningham's dance was an exponent of holy theatre in that what he saw in Cunningham's dance was simply his total absorbing of the moment of dancing unconcerned with what the dance itself may mean apart from just that (2008, p. 64). For us to appreciate Cunningham's dance, we need to shift our perception a little: we need to watch dance as if for the first time. Dance in Cunningham's conceptualization is like pure consciousness – thinking through each of the movements at a time from where the entire dance hence unfolds. There is discipline and there is technique as well as mathematical counts, and yet ultimately it comes down to the fact that dance is thinking with one's body. In dance, the mind unfolds as the visible trace of time, which is an underlying philosophical concern of Cunningham's entire work first explored in his seminal *Walkaround Time* (1968) which we will consider now.

Composed as a homage to Marcel Duchamp's *Large Glass* (1915–23) Merce Cunningham's 1968 premiere of *Walkaround Time* explored dance and its relationship to movement and time. For Cunningham, dance – as he suggests in the quote above – manifests a visible action of life. What do you think he means by that? In order to understand how dance relates to the sun coming up, it is perhaps helpful for us to first consider Duchamp's idea of the *ready made*. Marcel Duchamp (1887–1968) was a French-American painter, sculptor and ardent player of chess who created art works such as the famous *Fountain* (1917) – a urinal put upside down – by finding objects and placing them into a museum context to radically question society's perspective on art. He worked on *The Large Glass* for almost twenty years, first beginning his elaborate notes and conceptual studies which informed the work and were later published as *The Green Box* (1934). Also known under the lengthier title *The Bride Stripped Bare by Her Bachelors, Even*, the work combined intricate physical studies with the idea of eroticism as a mechanized process whereby the Bride apparatus in the upper panel related to the nine malic moles or bachelors in the lower panel next to the chocolate grinder apparatus.

The idea to reconstruct *The Large Glass* as the set for Cunningham's *Walkaround Time* emerged over a game of chess, when visual artist Jasper Johns first proposed the idea to Merce Cunningham sitting next to Marcel Duchamp and John Cage who played the game (Brown, 2007, p. 501). Since Cunningham shared a similar aesthetic sensibility and Duchamp was not opposed to the idea under the condition that

Johns would do the work of reconstruction, the creation of the dance was happily agreed. Intrigued by Duchamp's selected everyday objects, Cunningham's dance can be seen as a ready-made in the way that every single movement we observe in the world or choose to create ourselves can become part of the dance. Brown discusses that in fact there are many subtle references to Duchamp throughout *Walkaround Time* (see Brown, 2007, pp. 501–502). For Cunningham, dance thus postulates an existential given asserting that movement permeates all life, more or less in line with the world around us, chance-based and misleadingly unstructured at first glance – yet for the choreographer to think through and create subtle shifts in our perception of such synchronicity. As Deborah Jowitt describes Cunningham's dance to us:

> The subject, then, is life's processes, not tableaux and gestures from a particular life. And it is the ways in which he has attempted to bring his processes in line with his understanding of nature's "manner of operation" that make his dances and his dancers look the way they do. (1988, p. 282)

Cunningham's choreographic quest reoriented ballet and modern dance according to an analytic perspective of investigation, which rearranged movement material in line with the anatomical predisposition and movement potential of the body. His desire was not for the body to express or represent a narrative or concept, but rather for the dancer to be fully present to the precise moment of each movement itself. In her recent homage to Cunningham, Susan Foster points out how the attempt was not to synthesize ballet and modern dance, but rather to create a form of bricolage. She recalls,

> The technique brought together a barre-like set of introductory exercises for warming up and activating parts of the body, performed in the center of the room without the assistance of a barre; followed by the lengthier phrases performed in place and then traveling across the room. The exercises, executed both in parallel and turned-out positions, featured unusual pairing of arm, leg and spine movements, almost as if the dancer were conducting an inventory of possibilities. (2010, p. 7)

Cunningham's technique thereby initiates his dancers to access the invisible dance their bodies can articulate once that they are freed from the constraints of narrative expression. In "The Function of a Technique for Dance" (1951), Cunningham further explained how human movement is hardly a natural process per se, but rather a conscious intellectual effort to undertake.

Hence, the dancer's art process "can take actions of organization from the way nature functions", but Cunningham also stresses that these are "essentially man invent[ed] process[es]" (Harris, 1997, p. 60). Therefore, only through rigorous training and technique can "the final synthesis" be achieved, which is "a natural result, natural in the sense that the mind, body and spirit function as one" (Harris, 1997, p.60). Cunningham's point here is decidedly anti-balletic despite using certain techniques of that vocabulary. Thus his credo to anti-virtuosity proclaims that it is important "Not to show off, but to show; not to exhibit, but to transmit the tenderness of the human spirit through the disciplined action of a human body" (Harris, 1997, p. 60). The function of his technique is therefore to help access and channel life's moving energy rather than display a virtuosic formula. As Cunningham explains,

> Technique is the disciplining of one's energies through physical action in order to free that energy at any desired instance in its highest possible physical and spiritual form. For the disciplined energy of a dancer is the life-energy magnified and focused for whatever brief fraction of time it lasts. In other words, the technical equipment of a dancer is only a means, a way to the spirit. (Harris, 1997, p. 60)

Through daily practice, Cunningham dancers become experts at an ongoing exploration of movement potential to help them channel different levels of energy. Merce Cunningham's focus on technique – as that of many other choreographers in fact – is thus based on the dancer's intimate awareness of embodied modes of knowledge as the base of creativity and artistic freedom. The emphasis on dance's relationship to life-energy and spirituality is particularly important to stress in a context, where life itself could be extinguished instantly in the event of a nuclear war. Dancers were thus participating in a peaceful resistance that by withholding literate meaning created an experience not unlike meditation practice whereby perceptual conventions were disturbed so that a new awareness of time and space could emerge. Just as Marcel Duchamp could recognize beauty in everyday objects to revalue life and in particular the industrial manufacturing of utilities into commodities, Cunningham declared the dancer an independently moving spiritual source of movement energy and creation. The impulse is radically liberational but affords a spectator to go along on the dancer's journey and not get lost in his or her own conceptual preconceptions of what a dance is.

Cunningham's choreographic approach to dance was therefore concerned foremost with the rhythmical composition of the body in space and time. Investigating time, in particular, drew the line not only to Albert Einstein's (1879–1955) notion of space and relativity, but also to the continuity of structural phrasing of movement and energy which is at the heart of Cunningham's choreography. As a time-based art form dance – as time's moving image – is close to a Platonic notion of eternity and the transcendental. Cunningham argues with reference to the quote from Plato's *Timaeus*: "Time is the moving image of eternity" (in: Harris, 1997, p. 61). He thereby reinforced a cosmological link to the spiritual dimension of dance in line with his exploration of Zen Buddhism at the time. To quote Deborah Jowitt again, time as composed in Cunningham's choreography adhered to different parameters than were expected by dance audiences then:

> Time for the Cunningham dancer is not time as we associate with traditional theatre and music. Events do not develop over its passage, lead inexorably toward climaxes and die away. The causality of Newtonian physics has been abandoned for a more discontinuous reality. Climaxes, which Cunningham has disapprovingly termed "privileged moments," seldom rise from the web of events. Relationships between dancers may occur fugitively, but, although they may seem tender or playful or contentious, they are not fraught with evolving drama. (1988, p. 287)

Cunningham's work examines time from the moving perspective of the body: what can it do in how many different ways? The dancer is almost like a movement-machine or marionette, but at the same time undoubtedly human in the sweat and effort he or she spends to achieve movement precision and variation.

This is also made visible during the intermission, when dancers appear in their sweatpants and bathrobes to sit and stretch, wiping the sweat off their foreheads. The mundane is highlighted in ironic juxtaposition with the sung opera. There is no overt drama or action, no passions are revealed through the power of dance, but rather a cool, self-effacing seriousness that resists the temptation of emotive expression (see Copeland, 2004, pp. 25–51). By withholding narrative, the choreography forces the spectator to focus on the mechanisms of perception as such. Cunningham's dance aligns with Merleau-Ponty's phenomenological approach that we looked at earlier, but also relates to ideas of time and duration we considered with regard to Bergson's philosophy of time and image. Perceptually, it is up to the spectator to establish the possible relations between the separate entities of choreography for movement, sound and scenic composition. Only if we participate actively can we understand that the apparent "randomness" makes time transparent as the mere accumulation of simultaneous movements and sounds next to found and rearranged objects. *Walkaround Time* stages the dissection of "mind-time" by alluding to human consciousness and how it relates to synchronicity of movement that constitutes its own environment and meaning each instant.

The already mentioned affinity to Zen Buddhism that Cunningham shared with his lifelong collaborator and partner John Cage is all too evident (see Cage, 2004). As Carolyn Brown has described the connection to Duchamp's *Large Glass* and "stillness" in the work:

> "Still" is the operative word. Slowly, really really slowly, the right foot tentatively lifts off the floor with little pulsing developpés ending in a full developpé to fourth front, then held there hip level, balanced and absolutely still. [...] Out of this balanced stillness, I had to find the resources to immediately move fast and big, to take to the air, to cover space, and then return once again to absolute stillness and repose [...] Serenity and stillness, inner calm and outward clarity – these, I discovered, were the demands I needed to meet in *Walkaround Time*. (2007, pp. 504–505)

Even in the 1973 film version that exists, such stillness is conveyed that one has to be absolutely with the intricate detail of the movement to grasp the intensity of the work as well as its humorous note. The simultaneity of David Behrmann's soundscape "For nearly an hour" next to the dispersed choreography of dancers facing different directions at the same time, demands that we accept the dance for what it is: movement in space. The timeframe is thereby altered to an experience of almost timelessness: a pose could be seemingly held forever or shift unexpectedly.

Returning to Duchamp for a minute to see the relation between his art and Cunningham's choreography, it is said that in the *Large Glass* Duchamp attempted to blend sexuality with transition, and that the movement of machinery resulted in a combination of visceral and mechanical forms as to "metamorphos[e] painting into the living structures of the twentieth century" (Mink, 2000, p. 41). Stripped down to the fact of continuous movement, Merce Cunningham managed to reveal the power of dance as the moving image of time. However, time is of course the manifestation of life's moving energetic source or organic essence to recall Jerzy Grotowski's terms: atomic particles bouncing off each other, creating shapes and patterns that ultimately dissolve and recreate again. Thus, underlying the abstraction of Duchamp's *Large Glass*, we find life and eroticism at its creative source. As Duchamp described,

> Eroticism is a subject very dear to me, and I certainly applied this liking, this love to my Glass. In fact, I thought the only excuse for doing anything is to introduce eroticism into life. Eroticism is close to life, closer than philosophy or anything like it; it's an animal thing that has many facets and is pleasing to use, as you would use a tube of paint, to inject in your own production, so to speak. (Schwarz, 2000, p. vi)

The energetic life force therefore appears in many disguises in the mask of the artwork. From this perspective Duchamp and Cunningham merely dance on the other side of the expressive spectrum, where they have transcended the visibility of their form to target the invisible source of their creativity. As art historian Arturo Schwarz has pointed out with reference to the notion of mysticism in Duchamp's work, "Like all myths, this one too involves the use of an allegoric and a symbolic language in which puns and metaphors disguise the real content, accessible only to the initiate" (Schwarz, 2000, p. 84).

By analogy, Cunningham's choreographic approach transpositioned ballet and modern dance in order to express anti-hierarchical sentiments of the 1960s which opposed the centre perspective of ballet as well as the mythification of male–female relationships prevalent in the modern dance of Martha Graham and José Limón. By contrast, Cunningham's analytic approach towards movement sought to establish a perfect equilibrium among his performers on stage: a state of disengaged equanimity and repose. His aesthetics thus strongly reverberated with developments in physics during the late 1940s and early 1950s, where new cosmological theories developed around the notion of relativity and nuclear physics. As Adam Frank in his book *About Time* (2011) describes this perceptual shift:

> The synthesis created a new kind of cosmological theory describing the detailed evolution of space, time and matter. [...] Like an exquisitely choreographed ballet, all the known particles played their role on a space-time stage described by an expanding universe of general relativity. Each species in the subatomic zoo mixed with others and with particles of light (photons) in the ultrahot, ultradense primordial soup. Particle populations remained in perfect equilibrium, changing back and forth from one form to the other, until the cosmic expansion cooled and thinned the soup. (p. 194)

It is easy to think of Cunningham dancers as such "particles of light" or "species in the subatomic zoo" as they organize themselves in space according to a choreographic pattern that is chance-derived and perpetually changing just as evolution itself. After all, Cunningham choreographed it at a time when the big bang theory was first discovered and scientists hypothesized the early universe as a "nucleonic dance" of continuously moving and metamorphosing particles (Frank, 2011, p. 195).

In tune with the prevalent agnosticism of his generation, Cunningham was therefore not so much interested to reveal archetypal truths of the body or human experience but explored the relationships that result from a scientific approach towards analysing movement and what the body can do with the given elements of ballet and modern dance to move beyond the illustrative representation of myths and narratives. By the end of the Second World War it appears that the art world had finally come to accept that final truths could not be known and that all art could do was to question the status quo by resisting its representation. In that vein, Cunningham's dancers disengaged from overt political action and focused on the here and now of the act of dancing: being with it, rather than making any claims whatsoever about the significance of dancing in relation to the outside world. You can see how this is perhaps another way to stage civil disobedience, as one simply disengages from the political and becomes drastically resistant to a politics

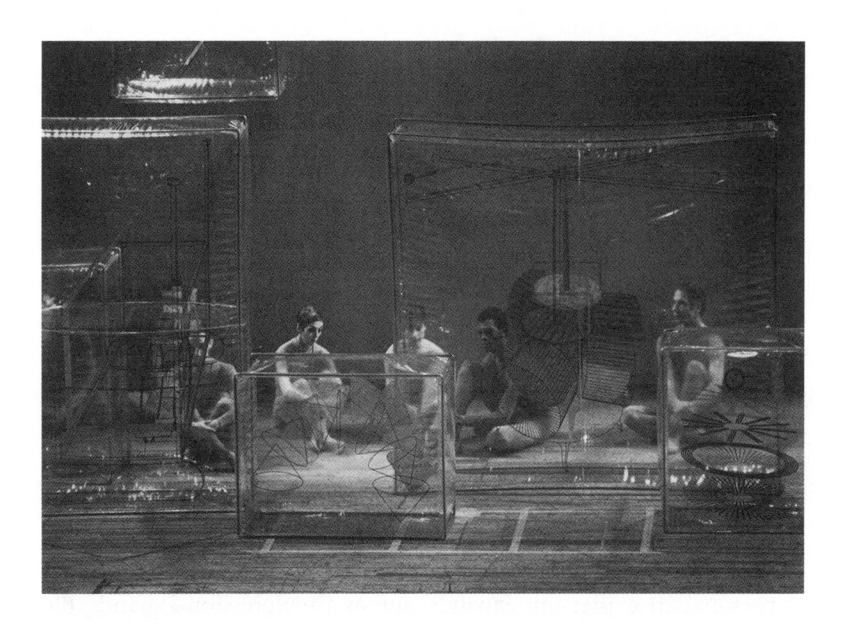

Merce Cunningham and Dance Company, *Walkaround Time* (1968)
© Photo by Oscar Bailey.

of violence based on ideology, power and representation. As a matter of fact, could we not say that nothing could have been more political at that time than doing just that: dancing in a world that was preoccupied with social upheaval, the Vietnam War and threat of nuclear extinction by either of the two world powers?

Body-space and task-based performance in Anne Halprin

Whereas Cunningham's quest was guided by the Zen-Buddhist contingency of the I-Ching, Anne Halprin found similar inspiration in the Californian natural environment outside on her dance deck. In comparison to Cunningham's post-Graham "aesthetic of indifference" (Roth, 1977, pp. 46–53), Halprin introduced a more overt contemporary ritualism as she "recast dance as a vital agent for community expression and social change" (Ross, 2007, p. 302). Her path led from "investigations of the structural logic of movement, to task performances" and eventually "ritualized group encounters, in which she began experimenting with dance as a way of healing society" (Ross, 2007, p. 302). Influenced by Gestalt therapy Halprin investigated "imagistic language" through which she claimed that she was "receiving messages from an intelligence within the body, an intelligence deeper and more unpredictable than anything" conceived rationalistically (see Ross, 2007, p. 305). Halprin's choreographies of psychokinaesthetic visualization thus created a movement-based form of physical therapy to amend not only the alienated teenage soul in 1960s America but also to help her fight cancer later on in her career. Her choreography ventured into the anthropological realm as to celebrate the continuum of the life/art process. As Janice Ross in her biography on Halprin describes,

> This method of working with dance seeks to access the life story of each person, and then use this life story as the ground for creating art. This is based upon the principle that as life experience deepens, personal art expression expands, and as art expression expands, life experiences deepen. (2007, p. 318)

In 1968/69, Anne Halprin choreographed *Ten Myths* as a series of participatory events in mutual creation with her audience-participants. Her intention was for her "[a]udiences [to] create their own spontaneous links between their psyches and an invented vocabulary of movement symbols" (Ross, 2007, p. 224). These were performances in the style of contemporary "mini-rituals", which blurred the line between real life and theatrical experience. Environments were varied for each event according to their theme and intention. For *Maze*, for example, she worked with a "12 foot high labyrinth suspended from a wire grid [which] was constructed from wrapping paper, newspaper and sheets of black, white and clear plastic" (Worth/Poynor, 2004, p. 21). Halprin combined these environments with "simple physical scores", which she intended to be "self-generating" (see Worth/Poynor, 2004, p. 21). Participants were thus challenged to alter the environment which they engaged with. In this case, for example, tasks were given in order to question the participants' relationship to contemporary media representations of the Vietnam War and 1960s political upheaval so that they would create and become their own embodied environment. As Libby Worth and Helen Poynor have characterized the impact of this work:

> Halprin's task in Myths was to create scores which gave individuals the freedom to respond in their own way to the stimulus offered, while providing a strong and flexible enough structure to facilitate the creative engagement of the whole group and to generate a sense of ownership. In her role as director Halprin responded to what was happening in the moment, modifying scores, introducing new ones or integrating suggestions from participants. Myths were in every sense "live" events. The transformation from "performance" to participatory event demanded an equivalent transformation in the role of the artist, from controlling artistic genius to creative facilitator and collaborator. (2004, p. 22)

Evidently, Halprin was particularly intrigued "to reengage the gestural vocabulary of everyday life as art and to cast the spectator as a more active participant" (Ross, 2007, p. 161). By breaking away from cause-and-effect linear narratives, yet remaining close to everyday experience and repetitive structures, her audiences were integrated as much as disoriented by the new aesthetic which swept not only newfound theatrical spaces from garage to public park but also influenced and acted against oppressive politics on the streets and in Vietnam.

Halprin's dance choreography and creative vision blended easily into the time of 1960s political activism discussed in the previous chapter. "Doing something" became the slogan of dance as much as street politics. In his influential "Bodies on the Gears Speech" (1964) available on YouTube, Mario Savio had first called for a student uprising to put their bodies on the line in order to demonstrate against state violence and protest the corporatization of university education and all other aspects of life. Also, Irving Goffman (1922–1982) had published his *Presentation of Self in Everyday Life* in 1952 a good ten years earlier which was enthusiastically received by dancers, performers and theatre practitioners of the day. Compared to Martha Graham's Jungian rituals of the Western psyche we discussed earlier, Halprin's concern for myth and ritual differed, as she took a more sociopolitical approach. Ross explains, "Ann's *Ten Myths*, in contrast, sought a new set of natural behavioral codes to replace cold war America's emphasis on containment, blind obedience to the government, and a materialist, middle-class life" (Ross, 2007, p. 234). In 1967 Richard Schechner published Grotowski's teachings on poor theatre with the *Tulane Drama Review* so that his aesthetics became more widely known. As many in her generation, Halprin also started to experiment with audience participation to get people politically involved and break down the distancing strategies of the proscenium stage. The 1960s are therefore often described as an aesthetic era of democratic "making rather than taking meaning" (see Perloff, 1991) which redefined spectatorship from merely visual towards a primarily tacit, embodied-experiential pleasure of actively taking part in performance.

Audience attention was significantly shifted towards "information within and without oneself and one's body, one's world" (Ross, 2007, p. 242). Modern dance teachings' legacy to the 1960s was therefore a continued "quest for a moral and democratic ideal" to be expressed "via the dancing body" (Ross, 2007, p. 242). From today's perspective, Halprin's essentialist trust in the inner truth of experiencing movement and dancing as vehicle to ecstatically turn the inside out matched a similar desire in method acting of the time, where being present and authentic within a character was the prevalent paradigm. As a member of Halprin's Dancers' Workshop, her daughter Daria Halprin, for example, testified to such astounding and yet somewhat naïve "wedding of emotions to actions while biasing the nonverbal" in her performance in Antonioni's 1968 film *Zabriskie Point* (Ross, 2007, p. 247). Striving for the communal experience, nude performances as Halprin's *Bath* (1967) attempted to break down the social mask to arrive at a "non-matrixed" presence via "tasks [which] did not create a fictional illusion of character and [...] existed in an actual, not imaginary, time and place" (Ross, 2007, p. 254). The ordinary and everyday emphasized the gestic in a Brechtian approach of supra-naturalism as Ross describes,

> By focusing on what is there in a ritual practice, like sitting still on chairs at a table and manipulating utensils to eat, one can see what isn't there, the invisible 'rules' behind these actions. Manipulating these rules can then become the basis for turning life actions into performance gestures. (2007, p. 263)

In the context of 1960s political upheavals, the previous chapter already discussed that theatre and dance artists of the time appropriated ritual in Victor Turner's broadest sense of communitas, as Anne Halprin's choreography of those years also testifies. Space, time and audience were exposed to ritual as a means to access practical self-knowledge and societal change. Rhythm, movement and kinaesthetic experience were the essential ingredients that dance put into the political mix to make this change happen.

The RSVP cycle and creative process

In her later work, Anne Halprin focused on developing movement as a mode of life experience and healing that is now taught as part of the Tamalpa arts and therapy approach. Her movement ritual thus evolved as a sequence of movement explorations that focus on inner sensing, balance and breathing to raise kinaesthetic awareness and expression (see A. Halprin, 1995 and Worth/Poynor, 2004). Unlike a fixed dance technique, this approach allows for authentic movement expression to occur as it relates to the individual's anatomy and psychology. Halprin refers to the emanation of such movement as "resource" which is then used as part of the "scoring process", "valuaction" and "performance cycle" she developed together with her husband Lawrence Halprin who pursued similar interests and concerns in architecture (see L. Halprin, 1969). Underlying both of their work in dance and architecture is the investigation of the "creative process", as it can be found in all human activity and cultural process with an attempt to channel creativity as a more holistic and organic approach addressing current environmental and ecological concerns (see Halprin, 1995).

In the ten-day workshop I took at Tamalpa in 2009 we were introduced to the basic principles of Movement Ritual I, scoring processes and RSVP cycle as well as a one-day exploration of performance work in the natural environment outside the dance deck and on the beach at Point Reyes, California. The initial attention placed on the spine and breathing is essential to open the body for physical exploration and kinaesthetic awareness. Halprin's teachings place different emphasis on all parts of the anatomy as they relate to human experience and feeling. Often, inner emotions and images are brought to awareness and allow individual experience and expression to emerge. The work is then shared with a partner, sometimes also with the entire group or may even find its way into a final performance. Lawrence Halprin's work in architecture explored scores in their many cultural functions from music to cooking, art and design where they manifest the human creative process. In continuation of the cultural revolution, their shared concern was for the environment and an ecological balance that protected life on the planet. Halprin's definition of dance was thus one step further removed from Cunningham's revolution, as her approach was rather more organic than technical. Movement related directly to the human soma and psyche, for Halprin there was no separation between the two. In that sense, her concern for space was always social and deeply

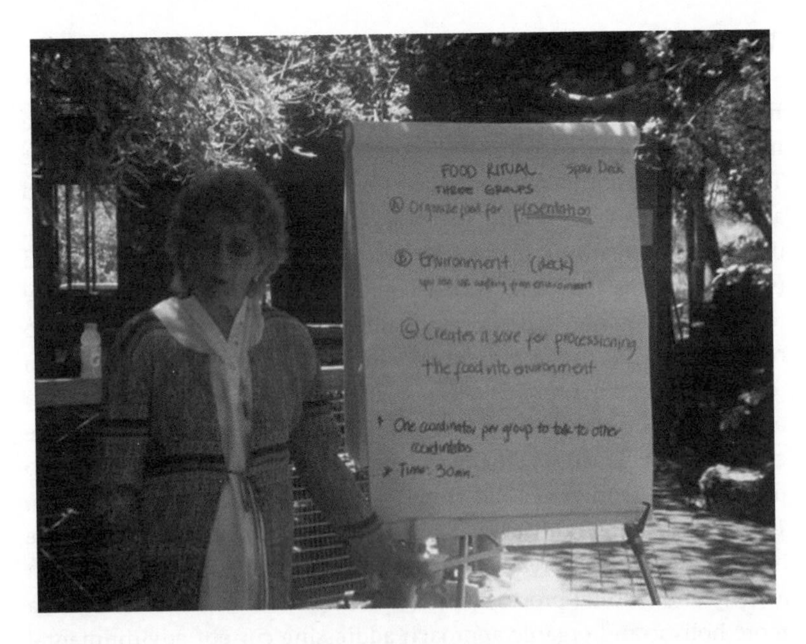

Anne Halprin, Tamalpa Workshop 2009 © Sabine Sörgel.

involved in community work rather than bringing dancers close to moving objects in an exhibition space. Her politics were always involved with people's lives and how to make them better as a teacher, choreographer and dancer. She was thus more involved in pedagogy than most of the practitioners we have looked at so far, and her influence on the generation to follow cannot be underestimated for that reason.

After the revolution: Yvonne Rainer's *Trio A* and the evolution of postmodern dance

Impressed, yet "not taken in", Yvonne Rainer further distilled the major elements of the American modern dance revolution to become one of the foundational members of US postmodern dance (Rainer, 1974, p. 372). While disconnected from the balletic sources of the Cunningham training, she focused on the elements of ordinariness and task-based crafting of movement he proposed – elements Rainer also strongly related to in Anne Halprin's work, when she and Trisha Brown took a workshop with her in 1960 (see Wood, 2007, p. 67 and Burt, 2006, pp. 55–56).

Together with Steve Paxton, Trisha Brown, Lucinda Childs, Robert Dunn and Deborah Hay, Yvonne Rainer pioneered the postmodern dance movement that united around the Judson Church from 1962 to 1964 (see Banes 1993 and Burt 2006). They shared with Merce Cunningham the neglect for Martha Graham's over-the-top psychologism and investigation of myth, yet were also increasingly critical of the discipline and demand Cunningham's technique placed on their bodies. Rather it was John Cage's chance principles as a mode of unintentional choreography they were intrigued by, as well as Halprin's engagement with tasks and scores developed outside the dance studio for the site-specific arena of public intervention. Aspects of movement vocabulary that they were interested in included pedestrian movement, contact improvisation and generally dance that countered any previous association with the form. Again, the body became their central focus point.

Yvonne Rainer, in particular, further developed Cunningham's exploration of energy by downplaying effort and phrasing. Her seminal *Trio A* was conceived as continuous movement without any climaxes or pauses thus counteracting the traditional convention whereby a dance was almost choreographed like a series of still photographs (Lambert-Beatty, 2008, p. 133). Unlike Halprin's authentic approach of gathering movement material, Rainer approached movement from a mechanistic, clock-work perspective: the dancer was regarded as a continuously moving engine downplaying volition and expression at all cost. Lambert-Beatty therefore describes Rainer's dance as decidedly "antiorganic" (2008, p. 139). Her interpretation of Rainer's *Trio A* thus suggests juxtaposing her dance and the mediatized images of the Vietnam War on American television (Lambert-Beatty, 2008, pp. 134–152). While television presented the death of people awkwardly near and distant at the same time – whereby in the worst instance you could simply switch off or move to the next channel or commercial – Rainer's dance solo in *Trio A* did not allow one to take any such pause as one movement led effortlessly into the next without a break or change of rhythm. On the other hand, Rainer asserted her body's "weight, mass, and unenhanced physicality" as a fact to be reckoned with (Lambert-Beatty, 2008, p. 152). *Trio A* was thus about the modulation of energy that dismantled dance conventions of her contemporaries Graham and Cunningham as she moved through them (Lambert-Beatty, 2008, p. 154).

To summarize some of the points raised in this chapter, Halprin and Cunningham spearheaded the movement towards postmodern dance during the 1960s. Their approach seemed to share some of the philosophical claims about the body and its ecstatic capacity to connect to the spiritual in the form of a creative transformation of physical energy towards levels of higher awareness of the body–mind continuum. Despite their stylistic differences in terms of dance vocabulary and choreography then, postmodern dance of the 1960s celebrated the body's political potential. Postmodern choreographers, in the wake of Cunningham and Halprin's pioneering efforts, sought to develop movement vocabulary beyond Graham-based psychological modernism in order to "find ways of generating movement outside the body", as Yvonne Rainer has phrased it and of course further developed in her own dance practice and task-based performances (Ross, 2007, pp. 149–150). So if we were to reconsider the word "task" in the context of the countercultural dance movement, it does not seem overly simplistic to ultimately reveal its perceptual shift towards dance as just another "ritual of human behavior", that is, movement as ready-made artwork.

Furthermore, 1960s American performance appears to be deeply embedded in the tradition of American pragmatism as, for example, Richard Sennet in his book *The Craftsman* (2008) points out. His analysis of craftsmanship observes how it has served as a tacit corrective based on experience, because it focuses on our direct, physical relation to the world and its objects around us. He continues to explain how current human experience under the conditions of global capitalism tends to negotiate between homo ludens, animal laborens and homo faber. Yet, it is work in the sense of labour, he argues, that capitalist culture values most to the unhealthy extent that it is seen as an end in itself rather than to reassert its playful, ritualistic function as facilitator for communal living (Sennett, 2008, p. 6).

Dance in the 1960s appeared to provide dancers with the skills to become craftsmen and women in their own right and was aesthetically very much in line with Cunningham's interest in technique or Halprin's task-based performances. As emancipated movers, these dancers indulged precisely in the physical exercise of repeated everyday movement practices, meaningful in their danced encounters, because they emerged from where technique and expertise in the form of cultural knowledge originally evolve (Sennett, 2008, p.9). As Sennett describes, "codes of honor become concrete by choreographing movement and gesture within the physical containers of walls, military camps, and battlefields on one hand, and shrines, burial grounds, monasteries, and retreats on the other" (2008, p. 12). In a way, he continues to argue, that the "craft of ritual [then] makes faith physical" and hence one finds the "philosophic issues embedded in everyday life" (Sennett, 2008, p. 14). Hence, dancers during this period developed their somatic skills to allow for a bodily connection to cosmological concepts of physical time and space as much as the natural environment through their kinaesthetic exploration of the world.

Lastly, these encounters may be perceived as "erotic" in terms of what Levinas has described in *Humanism of the Other* – namely, our moral obligation derived from our physical experiencing of pain and vulnerability. As Richard A. Cohen comments,

> One is moved to alleviate the pain of others because as an embodied being, the self enjoys the elements, is happy through them, and is thereby also able to appreciate viscerally the pain of physical suffering, deprivation, disease, and aging in others. (2006, p. xxxiii)

Looking at dance practices that emerged in the context of the 1960s counterculture, therefore, points to the grassroots political relevance of bodily practices. Whether these concerned the street politics and their speech act manifestations of non-violence or contemporary dance, kinaesthetic rituals appeared to physically contest the media footage of mass murder and dead bodies in Vietnam.

Study Questions:

1. What makes Merce Cunningham's approach of dance radical?
2. Cunningham, Halprin and Rainer had all trained with Martha Graham initially – can you still see traces of her influence in their work? Consider the importance of movement and how it relates to consciousness. What are the different aspects each choreographer emphasizes?
3. How does postmodern dance of the 1960s challenge conventional perceptions of time? What do you think were the political reasons behind this shift?
4. One of the major concerns next to time was space. How does site-specific work of the 1960s alter our understanding of theatre as "a place to watch" if we follow Greek etymology? Has it now become "a place to move" or even "dance"? Why do you think that is?

7 Unmasking the Social Mask in Post-War Tanztheater

Pina Bausch, Anne Teresa De Keersmaeker and Sasha Waltz

Made in post-war Germany: The dance theatre of Pina Bausch

Pina Bausch was born in 1940 in Solingen, a small town in Germany. She studied modern dance with Kurt Jooss at the Folkwang School in Essen which is known as the cradle of early twentieth-century expressionist dance in Germany. What was interesting about Jooss Ballet Company is that he was interested in the narrative structure of his dances – which he referred to as "dance dramas" – as well as socio-political commentary (see Schlicher, 1993). Jooss's renowned anti-war ballet *The Green Table* (1932) perfectly illustrates his approach, and Pina Bausch is known to have danced one of the leading roles in this piece. From 1960 to 1961 Pina Bausch received a scholarship to study dance in New York, where she took up classes at the famous Juilliard School of Music and studied ballet under Antony Tudor as well as modern dance with José Limón. Bausch returned to Germany in 1962 as solo dancer for the Folkwang Ballet and choreographed her first dance *Fragmente* four years later, when she became the company's director (Hoghe, 1986, p. 157). In 1973 she formed her own company in Wuppertal which was soon to become known as Wuppertal Tanztheater throughout the world. What was Bausch's secret?

Pina Bausch was born in the midst of the Second World War to become one of Germany's most acclaimed dance choreographers of the twentieth century. It is known that Bausch overheard the conversations of people gathering at her parent's local pub discussing the aftermath of war and fascism perhaps to find their way into the erratic tumbling of empty chairs in *Café Müller* (1978). Or so the story goes. While there is a degree of realism at the heart of Pina Bausch's choreographic process, it is such observational realism dismantled that makes her visual–kinetic world fascinating. More importantly, her choreography is held together by unrequited longing – called "Sehnsucht" in German– that binds her dancers together in a romantic quest for life's organic essence. Moments of suspended time insert themselves in a scenography of shared dreams. Sometimes tender, often violent, these visions articulate themselves in the movement choreography that abstracts and alters from the everyday vocabulary of our bodies in motion. As Janet Adshead-Landsdale summarized the impact of Bausch's repertoire of kinetic gestures:

> Gestures reverberate through the body, explicit enough to convey mood, but not so obvious to write a plot; sufficiently distinctive to invite speculation about narrative and relationship, but sufficiently ambiguous to avoid resolving it. Moments of wit are many – wit in movement (an exchange of dances), allusions to flying, swimming – but only half evident, barely stated. (Adshead-Lansdale, 1996, p. 21)

Founding her own company in the early 1970s, Pina Bausch revolutionized previous conceptions of dance, in particular ballet. She was less interested in the perfection of dance technique than in the investigation of the dancer's inner world. Indeed, Bausch, not unlike those other pioneers before her, was interested in the truthful revelation of the dancer's inner self by working through the fatal constructions of the social mask resulting in violence and war, and the many deaths as a consequence. In that sense, her quest did not consider how people move, but what moves them – as she has so often been quoted to say. She based her rehearsal technique on a set of questions for her dancers to create an improvisational score. For example, Bausch would give her dancers a theme such as childhood and ask them to share whatever associations in the form of a story or gesture would come to them working with the group. The material would then be gathered in a process similar to the editing of film images called "montage" (see Servos, 1998, p. 38). A way to describe Bausch's work therefore is episodic, but she also works with images that are derived from our cultural unconscious by working on ideas of mythology, the relationship between men and women, love, vulnerability, etc.

In Interviews, Pina Bausch often referred to the basis of her choreographic approach as based on a premonition derived from an intuition of movement that feels candid to human experience (Servos, 2008, pp. 229–245). When Bausch danced in *Café Müller*, for example, it was important that the gaze was consistently directed towards the ground, from where the source of the dancer's energy comes, even though or perhaps especially since her eyes were closed the entire time. With her bare feet deeply anchored in the ground, Bausch's movements appeared somewhat suspended and directed from those energies in the soil – not unlike the autumn leaves in *Bluebeard* (1977) later, which her then-partner Rolf Borzik had put on stage for Jan Minarek as *Bluebeard* to confront his archetypal double. In the video documentation of the performance – many of which were broadcast on German television during the 1980s – we can see how Pina Bausch's approach to dance focuses on small gestures, in particular the arms and hands that are always very elaborate in her choreographic work. For Bausch the whole body dances. Her repertoire includes a variety of everyday gestures, and you may want to recall Bourdieu's definition of habitus to describe how she points our attention and awareness to the cultural construction of these in manifestations of gendered stereotypes and clichés.

The fact that her dance theatre was screened on public television as well speaks of the impact her work received at a time when Germany was still recovering from the traumatic legacy of the Third Reich. To many people her work dismantled fallacies of society covering up the hidden violence that undermined families and relationships. Only in Bausch's later work of the 1990s into 2000s did her choreography become more intercultural and tender, and it seemed that some of the wounding had been redressed through her multicultural dance works and world touring. The later work as such speaks of an interesting shift the German society took after the fall of the Berlin Wall in 1989 by increasingly focusing on the European project and transnational identity, which will be looked at more closely with Sasha Waltz in the next section.

From the very beginning, Pina Bausch always worked directly with the cultural memories of her dancers who embodied diverse backgrounds in training such as ballet, modern dance or acting and was conveyed in their storytelling as a compositional choreographic tool. There is evidence of the rehearsal process for *1980*, for example, in which she would ask her dancers to recall motifs from childhood and make up movement improvisations on the grounds of those shared recollections. Dance music, like the waltz and tango with their laden social and emotional heritage, was also used as a backdrop for collective memories of archetypal memories and dreams. The movement repertoire hence consisted of small gestures emphasizing that the whole body can dance – in particular the hands and arms as a key Bausch signature. Bausch's use of habitual everyday movements deconstructed gender clichés through sheer endless repetition and variation. She constantly challenged her dancers to question themselves.

Norbert Servos, one of the first German dance critics to write about Bausch's dance theatre, characterizes the genre as "a total experience that allows the experience of reality in a state of sensual excitement" (1998, p. 39). If we were to compare Pina Bausch's work to Artaud, we would see how she emphasizes experience and mobilizes our affective memory and emotions. As Norbert Servos describes, her theatre is not "pretending", it "is" (1998, p. 39). Apart from this total engagement with her work, there are also several distancing devices that remind us of Brecht's use of scenic composition and gestus. For example, the principle of montage coupled with the stylized repetitions make us see an invisible truth behind the merely visible reality of these everyday gestures reminding us of Merleau-Ponty's notion that the body's meaning is constituted by lived experience. Radically present, Pina Bausch's dancing bodies evoke and re-inscribe archetypal gestures from the past – saturated as they are with childhood memories and cultural meaning – to form an artwork that transgresses such normativity of the real.

When sitting through a Bausch evening in the theatre, time is no longer measured by the clock, but the beat of your own heart. Enveloped by the energetic core energy – such as perhaps most evident in Bausch's *Rite of Spring* helped by the Stravinsky score – we find ourselves as an audience in the midst of all the social turmoil that surrounds us. Here we can feel how fascism and the two world wars start from the midst of our own wounded psyches. Peter Brook called this effect "holy" – the instance of recognition where the invisible-made-visible makes us see all the beauty and the terror of the human heart. Similar to what Peter Brook achieved in *Marat/Sade* by mixing Brechtian and Artaudian devices, Pina Bausch also uses choreographic gestus and affect as her ritualistic strategies to evoke deep emotional responses from her audience. By carefully inserting distancing devices such as the principle of simultaneity, however, we are never just swept away or overtaken by the emotion.

Here, Pina Bausch's work differs decidedly from her German predecessors Mary Wigman and Rudolf Laban who were both entangled with the Hitler regime for some time and fascist undertones have marred the image of German modern dance ever since (see Manning, 1993; Karina and Kant, 2003). Early modern dance and its affiliation with expressionism initially emerged as a counter-movement to the alienation of the early industrial age at Monte Verità, where Laban and his pupils founded an arts community to explore the potential of free movement, nudity and improvisation. This led to his more detailed analysis of choreutics and eukinetics as well as the Laban movement notation system later on in his life. Laban was drawn to Mary Wigman's emotional intensity as a dancer who expressed the deeper psychological split of the age in her early solo works such as *Hexentanz* (1926) and also her later explorations of choric dance forms. There is a tendency in early modern dance to dissolve the individual in the communal dance structure which has been interpreted as closely aligned to the Nazi propaganda machine of mass movement and mobilization as well as the fascist aesthetics and overt racism prominent in Leni Riefenstahl's film footage of the 1936 Olympics in Berlin. The fact, also, that both Laban and Wigman were invited to contribute choreography to the Olympics opening ceremony further underlines an affinity between fascist aesthetics and modern dance. Especially, the work of Wigman was considered somewhat anti-intellectual to the extent that her dances succumbed to a dark energy of choreographic works such as *Totenmal* (1930). Situated between the two world wars and the turbulent time of the Weimar Republic and ensuing Nazi terror, modern dance expressed the ambiguity around the question of the anonymous mass and community as well as the haunting of the many dead soldiers gassed in the trenches (see Toepfer, 1997). Pacifist pleas, such as the one most ardently expressed by Kurt Jooss's anti-war dance drama *The Green Table* (1932), were thus right next to the premonition of the demonic awareness of death and destruction looming underneath the layers of Western civilization.

Pina Bausch's dance theatre of the 1970s and 1980s picked up on this haunting legacy to the extent that her large ensemble of dancers on stage evoked a choric form and yet consistently deconstructed any attempt at false unification. A pupil of Kurt Jooss at Folkwang, Pina Bausch's early work is very aware of the dancer's kinesphere and orientation in space as well as the emotive intensity and gestural vocabulary she employed from everyday behaviours for narrative content and dramatic expression. Her dancers form a chorus, but within the chorus they always carefully maintain their individuality and expressiveness.

In her focus on "what makes people move" Bausch's dance theatre was first and foremost a theatre of experience (see Servos, 2008). An important aspect of her choreography is the use of space to evoke an emotional intensity for the audience directly derived from Laban's legacy as taught by his pupil Kurt Jooss. Anna Markard comments on the function of Laban's choreutics as choreographic tool:

> Choreutics is a tool for choreographic composition, for meaningful, communicative movement. The practise of Choreutics achieves discipline, co-ordination and sensitivity through awareness of gestural paths (trace forms) and directional focus through space. An understanding of the contrasting dimensional and diagonal directions stimulates the spatial imagination. Observation shows that there is also an inseparable relationship between human emotion and the direction of spontaneous physical action. A specific emotion will always favour a certain direction of directional path in space [...]. (1993, p. 50)

Choreutics play out in many ways throughout Bausch's oeuvre; however, unlike Jooss, Bausch's dance theatre works in a more surrealistic and elliptic manner. By using principles of filmic montage as a choreographic editing tool, her choreography allows for subtle emotional associations and witty repetition which reflected on unconscious impulses and motivations. Moving backwards from text and storytelling, Bausch's movement worked with energies that her audience could directly relate to and thus establishes a "sense of connection" which directly involves the audience "who are asked to question their interest and their own everyday experiences" (Servos, 1998, p. 37).

Bluebeard – While Listening to a Recording of Bela Bartok's "Herzog Blaubarts Burg" 1977

Pina Bausch's *Bluebeard – While Listening to a Recording of Bela Bartok's "Herzog Blaubarts Burg"* begins with a female dancer lying on her back and arms up in a frozen embrace. At the same time, a tall, bulky man in a black suit and long black overcoat sits contemplative on a chair in front of a moveable audiotape player. Both have bare feet – perhaps the only key initially that they are dancers – on a stage floor covered in autumn leaves designed by Pina Bausch's partner Rolf Borzik. The walls are washed down and are of clinical white with a tall ceiling and wide windows – a hall or rundown castle is referenced but could also be a prison wall. Initially, there is no sound as the man gets up from the chair with a blank expression on his face turning towards the lifeless woman lying on the floor covered by the brown leaves surrounding her. As he approaches, he suddenly bends down, unexpectedly swift – fulfilling a somewhat compulsive predicament to do so, and as she embraces his heavy figure on top of her slender frame, they both crawl backwards through the leaves. Yet, there is no escape. She opens her arms, and as the man is released, he turns back towards the audio-player for Bartok's opera to begin.

The opening sequence establishes the male–female dynamic that will structure the entire piece, as the man alias Bluebeard moves back and forth between the audio-player determining the scene and the solo dancer, Judith, grappling with her freedom. Their relationship is introduced as the frantic embrace of an overpowering male and a lifeless corpse trying to escape the compulsive repetition of their violent ordeal. The scene is slightly morbid because of the decaying leaves, and also the washed-down red nightgown garment Judith wears revealing her naked back. Her movements on the floor are constrained, tying her down, inhibiting her expression as she is fixed into static gestures. Crawling backwards on her back through the leaves, the dancer manifests a movement that signals an emotion of fear and strain, there is always tremendous effort and expenditure as well. At the same time, the movement is triggered as much as inhibited by the tall man seated at the tape recorder or lying on top of her in a position of power and dominance. The recurring movements during this sequence suggest sexual connotations and are sometimes of a violent force that can become tender, but always remains in an ambivalence, whereby the one can easily shift into the other.

Following on from the opening, Judith presents the other female dancers who she selects from the male and female chorus slowing walking in, holding hands, but with the heads bent down facing the floor. The posture they hold makes them appear as lifeless puppets, a cabinet of the dead rather than the living. Only the women Judith picks out – by taking their hand and lifting their heads – appear visible by presenting their face to Bluebeard and the audience. While Judith confronts Bluebeard directly with his single file of victims, the audience, too, becomes a witness to the scene. The archetypal myth is here confronted physically as the choreography responds to the violence of the musical score being stopped and played back at random. Instead of a dramatic logic, Pina Bausch presents the obsessive–compulsive repetition of a collective neurosis which places women at the whim of a male fantasy. However, Judith is not without agency in her manipulation of the events. She, too, directs Bluebeard's actions, propels him to start the tape again and look.

The women in Pina Bausch's *Bluebeard* wear their long, slick hair open and brush it over their heads with the torso hunched over, a semi-erotic gesture of self-abandon and yet almost evoking a degree of madness as the women will also sit down and pull their hair outward with extended arms like a tent. As Judith's alter egos, they have become discarded, abused or murdered presumably by Bluebeard himself or the other men who wear dark replica suits mirrored on his costume. The single-file disperses time and again, as the chorus of dancers dissolves into smaller clusters of alienated individuals, running across the stage and throwing themselves violently against the white washed stage walls of the figurative mansion. There is no escape from their historical fate. Only in the women's choreographed solos perhaps does their dance begin – initiating the typical Bausch movements of extended, elongated arms, reaching up and inward towards the body centre in a self-embrace, sheltering the female figure and yet inflicting a movement also reminiscent of self-harm turned inward that we find in *Café Mueller* as much as the earlier *Rite of Spring*. The female solo sequences reach out and draw back as the dancer exhausts herself in a battle against gravity and male force. Then, a moment of stillness. All dancers sit against the walls on all three sides their heads bent forward as in the beginning, exhausted – pausing – as the tape plays on. The audience witnesses an empty stage, brown leaves, a toppled chair and the moveable tape recorder at its centre.

Later on in *Bluebeard,* another prominent scene, when the men strip down and imitate the movements of body builders in front of a tiny plastic doll up stage – here the vocabulary is exaggerated and enlarged to a heightened naturalism that becomes ludicrous. The inversion through comic stylization suggests that the performance as such is unreal and that there is no female substance to the male fantasy and obsession. In *Bluebeard,* Pina Bausch reveals the archetypal plot of the violent male that seduces and kills women in his castle as a social construction of habitus founded on the repetition of violent acts and embodiments. The audience becomes a witness who fills in their own associations with culturally determined imagery and movement

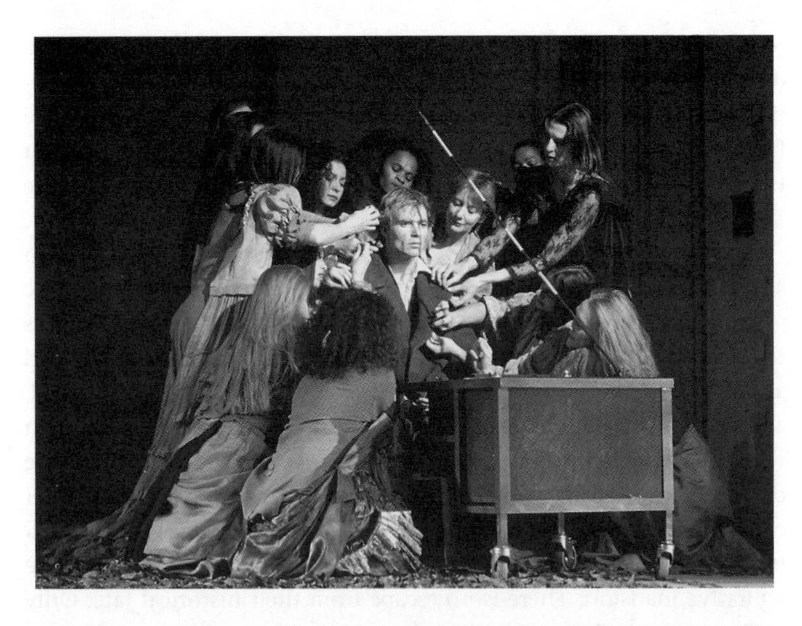

Tanztheater Wuppertal in Pina Bausch's *Bluebeard* 1993 © Bettina Stöß.

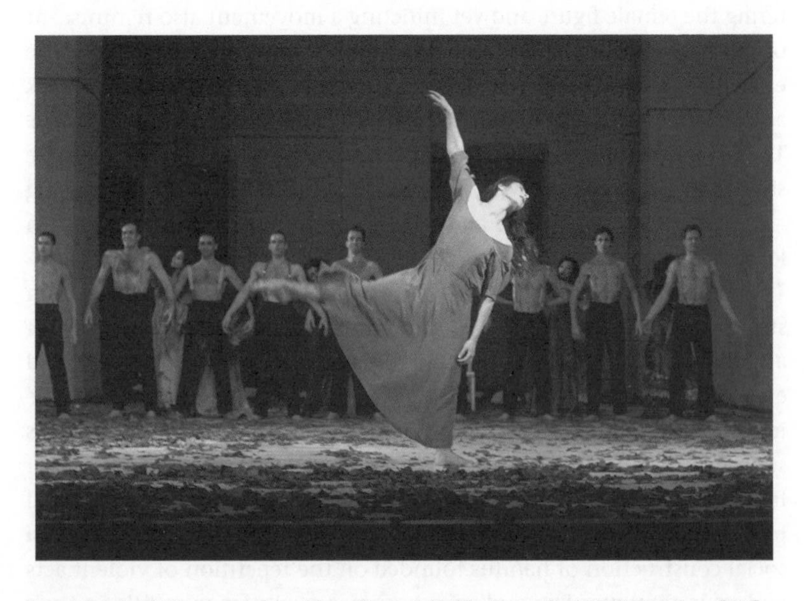

Tanztheater Wuppertal in Pina Bausch's *Bluebeard* 1993 © Bettina Stöß.

vocabulary; it makes them see and understand the social construction as to perhaps bring about change in response. However, Pina Bausch is never overtly didactic in her approach which is why we would find her hard-pressed to proclaim herself a feminist. The point seems to be less about the confrontation of men versus women, but rather posing the question as to why our interhuman relationships carry such ambivalent meanings and often disintegrate into violence rather than love which appears what most people long for after all.

Feminism and gender politics: From Pina Bausch to Judith Butler

In the 1970s Bausch's work was regarded as feminist, and she herself – although critical of feminism's confrontational politics – has said that "the themes are always to do with man-woman relationships, the way we behave or our longing or our inability, only sometimes the colour changes" (see Servos, 2008). Feminism of the 1970s as put forward by Luce Irigaray in 1977 when her *The Sex Which is Not One* (1985) was first published and critiqued how women would be represented either as mothers, virgins or prostitutes and how there was hardly any opportunity for them to break out of these rigid roles in the public perception. These stereotypes, feminists of the era argued, are largely manifested in language and the literary canon, novels, but also film and media. One way to make us conscious of how these gender roles are constructed is Pina Bausch's work in dance theatre, the other would be by finding new modes of writing from a feminist perspective.

More recently, Judith Butler's (*1956) theory on gender more clearly defined the performative nature of identity construction and feminist discourse. According to Butler, our gender identity is different from our biological sex in that it is mostly performed according to normative social standards and behaviours. Her theory picked up from linguistics and sociology combining J. L. Austin's (1911–1960) speech act theory with Bourdieu's notion of habitus as well as Foucault's analysis of discourse formation more widely. Discourse analysis and speech act theory go together in that both look at language and the objectified status of the body in Western society. While Foucault was primarily interested in the intersection of language and power, speech act theory would emphasize how language creates social facts and even changes in status, as for example a couple before and after the marriage vows. Butler's point was that gender unlike sex is based on what she conceived of as a "stylized repetition of acts", she explains,

> Gender ought not to be construed as a stable identity or locus of agency from which various acts follow; rather, gender is an identity tenuously constituted in time, instituted in an exterior space through a *stylized repetition of acts*. The effect of gender is produced through the stylization of the body and, hence, must be understood as the mundane way in which bodily gestures, movements and styles of various kinds constitute the illusion of an abiding gendered self. (1990, p. 140)

Butler was very interested in drag performances and how these have historically disturbed the normativity of gender in society. When Pina Bausch therefore dressed her male dancers in women's evening gowns, we see how her choreography created a similar effect, especially by repeating gendered movement sequences across both sexes.

Thus, Pina Bausch's women often wear long, beautiful ball gowns with wide openings on the back revealing the spine. They dance on high heels which they sometimes forfeit to the men in a comic gesture of cross-dressing. Comedy flips into melancholy as a man perhaps previously in a ball gown, later on eats spoons full of porridge for his mum and dad – as in the recent revival of *1980 Ein Stück* at Sadler's Wells in 2014. Bausch's dancers display the social habitus of the psychologically wounded generation that survived the Second World War by dismantling false power binaries as West German society slowly moved towards the reconciliation and internationalization of Germany as part of the European unification process of the 1980s and into the 1990s reunification process with East Germany as well. Her dancers came from all over the world and constituted a vision of the European Union as its political entity was in the making. Travel became one of the company's strategies and found its way into the later so-called intercultural choreographies and collaborations (see Elswit, 2013).

Dance theatre in Belgium: Anne Teresa De Keersmaeker (*1960) and the Flemish Dance Wave

Contemporary dance in Belgium virtually did not exist before the appearance of Anne Teresa De Keersmaeker on the international scene. Although Maurice Béjart drew large audiences for ballet as the director of La Monnaie, Brussels national opera, as well as through his internationally acclaimed school Mudra, contemporary dance – successful in the United States and beginning to take root elsewhere – was not yet heard of here. Not until the 1980s then did postmodernism fully arrive in Brussels (see Uytterhoeven, 2002, p. 298). Flemish dance stood out for its interdisciplinarity as it was promoted by the international festival culture installed by the Klapstuk Festival. As Rudi Laermans points out, the international festival scene introduced De Keersmaeker and others to the works of Merce Cunningham and Trisha Brown at the time (2011, p. 406).

Anne Teresa De Keersmaeker's debut as a choreographer was *Ash* which she premiered in the late 1970s. She had studied humanities and dance with Lieve Curias, a student of Jeanne Brabants at l'Institut Municipal pour le Ballet d'Anvers, and also Lilian Lambert through whom she met Michèle Anne and Thierry De Mey (Uytterhoeven, 2002, p. 298). De Mey first introduced her to the writings of Artaud and Bataille and encouraged her to listen to the music of Steve Reich and watch the German film-maker Rainer Werner Fassbinder (Uytterhoeven, 2002, p. 298). Her main ambition at the time was to audition at Mudra where she would study from 1978 to 1980 among Nacho Duato, Bernard Glandier and Nicole Mossoux (Guisgand, 2007, p. 15; Uytterhoeven, 2002, p. 298). She also studied at NYU's Tisch School of the Arts 1981 – when she wrote her article on Valeska Gert for *The Drama Review* – on a Belgium scholarship for one year. At that time she was able to see modern dance giants Martha Graham and José Limón as well as their postmodern offspring Cunningham, Childs, Brown and Paxton who were still dominating the contemporary dance scene in the United States (Uytterhoeven, 2002, p. 298; Guisgand, 2007, p. 18).

Upon her return to Belgium, De Keersmaeker was programmed for the Kaaitheater festival which coincided with a fruitful phase of theatre funding across different European countries at a political time when the European Union found itself still in its infancy (Uytterhoeven, 2002, p. 299). Dance appeared as a welcome ambassador of cross-cultural arts collaboration paving the ground for the opening of national borders and easier access to work across countries of the European Union. Among the contracted partner institutions are Théâtre de la Ville in Paris, Hebbel-Theater Berlin, Rotterdamse Schouwburg and Springdance Festival Utrecht in the Netherlands and also Festival D'Avignon and Brooklyn Academy of Music in New York City. Under

Gantois Gérard Mortier – as the new director of La Monnaie in Brussels – De Keersmaeker received the unique opportunity to showcase her new work on a regular basis (Uytterhoeven, 2002, p. 299). In 1992 under the next director, Bernard Foccroulle, De Keersmaeker's company *Rosas* became the resident company at La Monnaie. During this period, De Keersmaeker achieved three things: 1. to regularly produce choreography with live music, 2. to develop a repertoire with the company funded by La Monnaie and 3. the foundation of her own school PARTS in 1995 (Uytterhoeven, 2002, p. 299; Guisgand, 2007, p. 16).

Since then, *Rosas* has achieved wide international recognition and acclaim. Upon the company's twentieth anniversary, Michel Uytterhoeven gathered the following data to account for the company's success: beginning with *Fase* the company counted 71 dancers from 19 different countries who shared their personal stories and cultural influence as part of the credits to each choreographic work – not unlike Pina Bausch's ensemble in Germany at the same time (2002, p. 299). For over twenty years *Rosas* gave 1728 performances in 37 countries and 202 towns and cities. At the same time PARTS auditioned in 28 towns and cities in 21 countries on 3 continents. From 1995 to 2002 212 students from 37 different countries were selected to attend the school (Uytterhoeven, 2002, p. 299). The teachings included creative exchanges with William Forsythe, Pina Bausch and Trisha Brown bringing together stylistic elements from classical ballet, German expressionism and US postmodern dance in De Keersmaeker's unique blend.

Fase, Four Movements to the Music of Steve Reich (1982)

Fase, Four Movements to the Music of Steve Reich (1982) was De Keersmaeker's choreographic breakthrough after she returned from New York and became an instant international success. Between 1982 and 1985 alone, *Fase* ran over a hundred times all over Europe and in the United States (Guisgand, 2007, p. 23). The choreography is structured in four parts: *Piano Phase, Come Out, Violin Phase* and *Clapping Music,* and the dancers are Anne Teresa De Keersmaeker and Michèle Anne De Mey. The two dancers are identically dressed, and much of the fascination of the movement relies in its effective use of repetition and ever so slight variation to capture the audience's attention throughout. While repetition and variation were regarded the key elements of minimalism in the wake of Yvonne Rainer and the Judson school, *Fase* appropriated this technical devise of American postmodern dance to articulate a rather specific subjectivity at the heart of DeKeersmaeker's choreographic project. Guisgand, for example, reads the rotation around the dancer's body axis as the gathering of energy that surrounds the dancer as an expression of self that radiates but does not reveal anything but its self-referentiality: the body's subtle rotation around an energetic core (2007, p. 32). The same is true for DeMey dancing alongside De Keersmaeker in the existing film of the piece. Both dancers share a complicity which is indicated by the smirks and shared glances that we see on the film every once in a while, when the camera zooms in on a close-up of the dancer's facial expression. Their complicity appears to consist of a balancing act they perform between secrecy and disclosure – a mystery code they have devised and agreed for themselves in the rehearsal. Repetition and variation thus coexist on a compositional continuum that permeates their dancing and becomes the dance as an unfolding structure that is anchored in their agreement and yet freely performed throughout.

The second dance *Come Out* has both dancers seated on chairs below a lamp that creates the scene of an investigation. Here, the movements have a hard and staccato rhythmic quality focusing on gestural vocabulary around the upper torso and shoulders. The binary rhythm is constructed around the triangle of the head and shoulders in a rapid sequencing of repeated movements that tie both dancers to a limited form without visible context (Guisgand, 2007, p. 27). At the same time, the audience listens to the interrogation of a young black American as part of Reich's musical score highlighting the physical confinement placed upon the dancers by the hand circles they perform and footstools they sit on (Guisgand, 2007, p. 27). The discrepancy between abstract movement choreography and setting juxtaposed with the sound and context Reich provides leads the audience into a space of accumulation mirrored and deconstructed by the choreographic score. In a flash, one witnesses rather than interprets the confinement and dehumanization of mechanization and procedure executed in the dance as an abstraction of the oppressive social structure the musical score alludes to. More powerful than a mere illustration, the physical score thereby evokes a kinaesthetic response in the audience which subtly critiques the underlying political system by deconstructing embodied physical conditioning in the accumulation and repetition of oppressive movement sequencing.

Come Out is followed by Anne Teresa De Keersmaeker's solo *Violin Phase* focusing on one of her choreographic obsessions: the spiral. In the film version by Thierry De Mey she is outside on a plateau in the forest with her feet tracing circular pathways in the sand. Guisgand's analysis of De Keersmaeker's choreographic oeuvre has identified the spiral as a key choreographic motif she returns to in all of her dances (2007, pp. 29–30). In *Violin Phase* the spiral indicates perpetual movement as the crisis and apotheosis of circularity in the constant evolvement and return of the same pattern. Circles of footsteps and arms, circles of her rotating skirt and skipping legs, circles of the torso and head. The spiral propels outward and inward demarking a fundamental sense of outside and inside spatial awareness. The energy of the spiral is energetic-creative as it permeates the cosmos and all living forms.

As such the spiral symbolizes possible flights, shifting meanings and points of changing direction throughout (compare Guisgand, 2007, pp. 29–30). Sapir explains,

> In its simplest form, De Keersmaeker's spiral consists of two complimentary or opposing phrases of movement that influence each other. More generally, the spiral's manifestation in her work ranges from an actual pattern delineated on the floor to guide the dancers through a particular sequence in rehearsals, through the overriding principle according to which a certain piece is constructed, to the trajectory of relationships between individual works. (De Keersmaeker/Sapir, 2008, p. 29)

Consequently, De Keersmaeker's heightened minimalism in *Fase* consists in the double play of dance and music as dance movement is not merely an illustration or visualization, but rather incorporates the rhythmic patterns and complexities of the Reich score. As Reich commented years after *Fase* premiered, De Keersmaeker's choreography completed his music to an extent that no one else had understood his work before (Guisgand, 2007, p. 32). Indeed, De Keersmaeker's choreographic starting point is almost always the music to which movement is created as an affective response (Burt, 2004, p. 36).

More recently, Renate Brauninger stressed how the affective intensity created by the minimalist score evokes a trance-like state (2014, p. 48). In her opinion an analysis of De Keersmaeker's work therefore needs to further reflect on the energetic shifts created by the work (2014, p. 49).

Steve Reich's music is similarly "fixed in its procedures, yet not quite fixed in its execution or playing out" (Brauninger, 2014, p. 49). As a compositional principle, Reich's music introduced "phasing", which Brauninger defines as "the constant repetition with slight changes" to create differences and variations in the audience's perception and attention (2014, p. 51). This transpositions into De Keersmaeker's choreographic process as follows:

> De Keersmaeker, like Reich, is interested in setting up and playing out preconfigured structures. There is a moment when the embodiment of the sparse movement material by the two dancers, and the sense they must have of one another as they dance together, asks for a "dancerly" engrossment analogous to that of the musicians when they engage with the phasing process in Reich's music. In both compositions, once the performers begin, they must place their concentration on one another in order to set in motion the processes intended by composer and choreographer. (2014, p. 52)

De Keersmaeker's work, so Brauninger suggests, zooms in on the affective-energetic qualities of the movement rather than its meaning (2014, p. 59). The trance-like effect De Keersmaeker's choreography creates collapses Western space-time sensibilities as the movement repetition evokes a sense of timelessness and transcendence (Brauninger, 2014, p. 61).

Guisgand describes this relationship in more detail, when he comments upon the aesthetic effect of this strategy for the spectator. Almost paradoxically, music and dance create a temporal parathesis which places the spectator into a perceptual abyss or trance as interpretation is replaced with timing and rhythm. As spectators, we are not so much asked to think but to be fully present to the dance which itself alters in movement as it creates its form as physical expenditure (Guisgand, 2007, p. 31). Moreover, De Keersmaeker breaks with the traditional audience gaze and expectation denying any pleasure derived from mere virtuosity as it is coupled not with narration but rhythmical complexity and intensity that affects the spectator's own energy field. Dancers and spectators are thus set free in a mutual game of structural composition and endless variation (compare Guisgand, 2007, p. 59).

Fase ends with the final part called *Clapping Music*, another duet created by De Keersmaeker and Mey – this time standing and skipping upright under the lamps from the previous *Come out*. As both dancers are still wearing the same white sneakers and outfit, the section repeats some of the gestural movement in an inversion of the previous section. To Guisgand this final section epitomizes De Keersmaeker's aesthetic as distinct from both the American postmodern as well as German expressionist school (2007, p. 31). He argues that the two dancers' self-effacing, almost neutral, performance exposes them in profile without any variation to an extent that evokes transparency, and yet the inner energy they both mobilize to perform the dance is immense. The question De Keersmaeker poses here is that we consider how the interplay of body, emotion and structure either constitute or more likely withhold meaning. In a way, this radical approach puts her right in the middle of postmodern formal purism and expressionist emotional expenditure (Guisgand, 2007, p. 31). Seeing *Fase* in 1992, dance critic Nadine Meisner had the following to say:

> To see *Fase* again is to re-experience the shock of youthful daring. As a hymn to minimalism it may be of its time, but it also transcends time; De Keersmaeker and Michèle Anne De Mey still perform the piece, looking only a little older but just as compelling. Like the music, the three duets and the solo each have their own narrow language and resonance, not only matching but enriching Reich's procedures through simple movement, reiterated, modified and accumulated. (Meisner, 1997, p. 11)

Following her analysis, De Keersmaeker's movement repertoire consists of small gestures "buil[t] into elaborate phrases that are exhaustively reiterated and then shift into something else" (Meisner, 1997, p. 12). Dancers often perform in counterpoint and change from abstraction to expression (Meisner, 1997, p. 12).

Rosas danst Rosas, a film by Thierry De Mey (1983)

The set of the *Rosas danst Rosas* film was an old school building, slightly dilapidated, constructed in 1936 by the famous Beligian architect Henri van de Velde. It is a three-storied U-formed architectural space built around a central playground with a complex internal structure, with long corridors and a lot of empty classrooms – often divided by

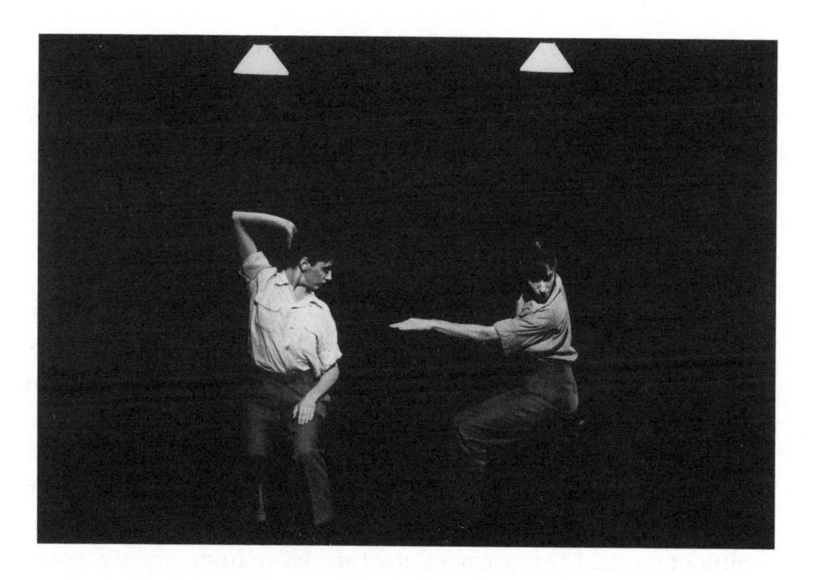

Anne Teresa De Keersmaeker's *Fase* © Herman Sorgeloos.

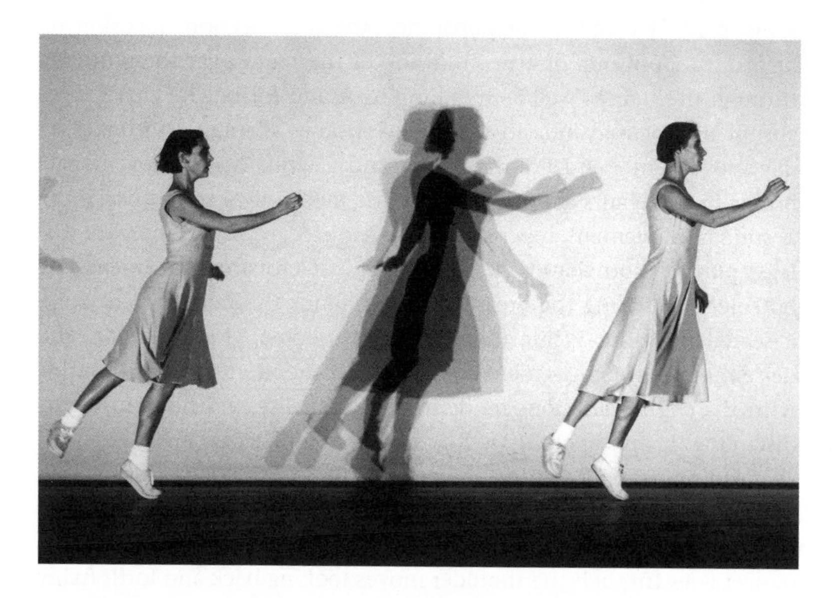

Anne Teresa De Keersmaeker's *Fase* © Herman Sorgeloos.

transparent partitions. The specific characteristics of the architecture, the transparency created by walls of glass and internal light shafts, are fully exploited by specific travellings and shots (see De Mey/Keersmaeker, 2002). Apart from the film itself, the DVD also contains the video documentation of the four movement sequences as developed and performed on the theatre stage:

> The score (composed by Thierry De Mey and Peter Vermeersch) of *Rosas danst Rosas* has four distintly separate parts, each of which is characterised by techniques of phasing, repetition and movement. The choreographic structure is defined within this framework. At first there is only movement on the ground, then on chairs. Next the space is explored and finally the whole "scene" is usurped in the fourth movement, a physical fight to finish which ends in a fifth part, a coda in which the dancers resume movements of each part without music. The movements used are drawn from everyday observations: the hand through the hair, looking to the side, propping the chin on the elbow, letting the head hang, falling, running ... (see De Mey, 2002)

Movements 1A and 1B demonstrated the floor section, focusing on breath, propping up of arms, running of the hand over the skull and through the hair as well as spiralling back and forth. The changes are abrupt and focused and most of them appear as adaptations from every day movement (see De Keersmaeker and Cevijik 2012). Movement 2 brings in the chairs accompanied by the mechanical sound backdrop; a similar movement repertoire is developed by using more of the legs, putting both hands between them, or crossing and uncrossing both legs, touching the breast, running hands through hair etc. from a seated position. While these appear gendered, the repetition also de-semiotizes the movement so that it becomes a mechanized routine with the slight variations rendering individuality and humour to the discipline. It appears that De Keersmaeker emphasized affect as much as meaning using the different energy centres of the body throughout. This is particularly evident in movement 3, where three dancers keep whirling (a familiar movement sequence from *Fase*), while the solo dancer goes through the shoulder moves looking back and forth fixing the gaze of the audience and finishing with a mischievous smile. The last section on the DVD is movement 4 with all four dancers moving in the diagonal (see De Mey, 2002).

Although many critics have read De Keersmaeker's work as concerned with gender, she herself regards her own choreographic process as more interested in structure (space and energy), rhythm and colour as was already discussed (1992, pp. 13–14). It appears that similar to Bausch's dance theatre, De Keersmaeker's critics emphasized the exploration of gender in the company's work of the 1980s, when originally De Keersmaeker included only women. However, De Keersmaeker herself – also not unlike Bausch – always resisted that reductive interpretation from the dancer/choreographer point of view which was more interested in the exploration of movement, time, space and energy. When she included men in *Achterland* (1990), it became apparent that her choreographic interest was to insert a further variant as to explore themes of bodily similarity and difference as well as different qualities of energy (Meisner, 1997, p. 12). Sapir comments,

> De Keersmaeker is interested in such non-Western traditions and very ancient dance forms, in which structure and expression come together. She is indebted to Taoist thinking which sees the division between structure and expression as inappropriate, believing that they are merely different manifestations of energy. Accordingly, she uses structural systems to think about such fluid concepts as energy and dynamics. (Sapir, 2008, p. 3)

It therefore appears that while we can read meaning and gender into the work, the work itself does transcend too facile an interpretation, or alternatively we may also say that the dance itself is larger than the personification embodied by the dancer.

Sasha Waltz's *Body Trilogy*: German dance theatre from the 1990s into the new millennium

A phenomenon of the post-wall Berlin republic, Sasha Waltz's dance theatre of the 1990s introduced a new aesthetic of dance realism that was initially also reminiscent of the grotesque aesthetics of Weimar variety and cabaret a la Valeska Gert – at least so it was received by some of the critics of the time (Schmidt, 2002, p. 338). Waltz's *Travelogue Trilogy* (1993–1995) and *Allee der Kosmonauten* (1996) – which portrayed the charming melancholy and slightly neurotic behaviour of an East Berlin flat share and made into prize-winning TV film in 1998/99 – were

Sasha Waltz's early international successes with her company she called Sasha Waltz & Guests. *Allee der Kosmonauten* presented a combination of slapstick realism and comedy where dancers would tumble over and off the living room sofa and pas-de-deux with the vacuum cleaner across the carpet. In 1999 Waltz became the co-director of the legendary Schaubühne alongside theatre director Thomas Ostermeier to succeed the legacy of Peter Stein's world-renowned ensemble. For a brief moment, dance and theatre came together under an aesthetic umbrella that was interested in the rediscovery of the body as the centre of a new theatrical realism spearheaded by the British wave of in-yer-face theatre first and foremost through the European reception of Sarah Kane and Mark Ravenhill. In a manifesto that announced Thomas Ostermeier's artistic vision for the new co-directorship with Sasha Waltz, dance and theatre work at the Schaubühne set out to work more collaboratively around a shared aesthetic endeavour to pay attention to felt pain and pathos as the mark of a new political realism that was supposed to counter postmodern deconstructions of the subject (Ostermeier, 1999, p. 13).

Sasha Waltz's *Körper* was the opening premiere and investigated aspects of the body in culture, anthropology, philosophy and architecture questioning such themes as the body's material essence(s), surfaces of skin and touch, as well as its capacity for narration and social ritual (see Müller, 2011, n.p.). As Berlin-based journalist Katrin Bettina Müller recalls the astounding takeover by the dancers as they confronted the vastness of the Schaubühne space:

> "Körper" was another homage to architecture commemorating this time the design of the Schaubühne – the former cinema built in 1927–28 by Erich Mendelsohn which remains one of the earliest examples of modern architecture on the Kurfürstendamm. Never before had the full height and length of the stage area been utilized in this way: the towering walls were reminiscent of a cathedral, the warmth of almost naked bodies contrasted with the coolness of bare concrete, both becoming pure embodiments of man and architecture. Part of the choreography involved the precise measuring of the stage area in terms of shoulder widths and back lengths; stacked bodies erected walls inside the room, marked its boundaries or divided it into separate segments. Taking possession of the theatre in this way, new images of our bodies' relation to space emerged – a subject not

often touched upon by dancers and choreographers but seldom in direct relations to a specific piece of architecture. (2011, n.p.)

The size of the Schaubühne space changed Waltz's perspective on choreography, and her work became increasingly more abstract as she moved away from the early social-realism of the earlier *Travelogue Trilogy* (1993–1995) and *Allee der Kosmonauten* (1996). Sasha Waltz's project thus marks the next generation of German dance theatre after Pina Bausch bringing a more somatically oriented approach in response to history and space to her choreographic process. While Sasha Waltz's first training in dance was with a former pupil of Mary Wigman in German expressionist dance, she also received training in ballet as a young girl and most significantly postmodern dance as a student at the Amsterdam School for New Dance Development.

Contact Improvisation and release technique are dance practices Waltz works with by emphasizing weight and gravity in a shift away from the central body axis. Movement improvisation appears as a strong foundation she has used to develop her own movement systems and motifs that reappear in the work over the past twenty years. Her interest in movement is almost physics-oriented as she choreographs her ensemble as a group interested in the interrelationship of mass and weight, each individual dancer becoming part of the larger whole reminiscent of moving particles in space. Touch, as in contact, was initially very important, and even if not visible in the end product any longer, it was an important phase of the rehearsal process and organic generation of the movement material (Schlagenwerth, 2008, pp. 41–47). Another important choreographic element is Waltz's dedication to explore the relationship between dance and architecture as her mode of practice-research in a series of workshops she calls "Dialogues".

The "Dialogues" are an integral part of her choreographic process and have continued as a practice alongside the performance work Sasha Waltz & Guests have produced over the last twenty years. Space is the central element for Waltz, who is the daughter of an architect, and who first thought of herself as a visual artist rather than a dancer/choreographer (Schlagenwerth, 2008, 14). In preparation for *Körper*, for example, Waltz pre-premiered material she first rehearsed at the independent venue Sophiensaaele which she and her husband, Jochen Sandig, had installed as one of the most successful independent theatre venues in Berlin-Mitte after reunification ("Dialoge '99/I"). Later on, this material was further refined during a six-week rehearsal process in the newly built annex to the Jewish Museum designed by the world-renowned Polish-Jewish architect Daniel Libeskind ("Dialogue 99/II"). Architecturally both of these venues are key memory sites that spatially embody German history before and after the Second World War. While the Sophiensaaele had been frequented by the political leaders of the Communist Party, Rosa Luxemburg and Karl Liebknecht, during the Weimar Republic, the Jewish Museum designed by Daniel Libeskind during the 1990s addressed German-Jewish history after the Holocaust from a distinctly postmodern-deconstructivist architectural sensibility.

Completed in 1999, the Jewish Museum was one of the first buildings constructed after the German reunification. Designed one year before the Berlin Wall came down, Libeskind conceptualized the building such that visitors to the museum would move along three underground axes of German-Jewish life commemorating the impossibility of disconnecting Berlin's present from its German-Jewish past. Thus the first axis is dedicated to the continuity of Jewish life and culture in German history, the second devoted to Jewish emigration and hope and the third to the Holocaust. Another layer to the building is the so-called spatial "voids" which mark the unspeakable atrocity of the extinction of Jewish life which Libeskind has referred to as representing "That which can never be exhibited when it comes to Jewish Berlin history: Humanity reduced to ashes" (2000, n.p.). The building as such is remarkable, because of the way that movement is spatially created as a parcours each visitor moves along. A visit to the museum thus becomes its own spatial-kinaesthetic experience that creates an affective-energetic response. The formal abstraction allows for a rather concrete personal experience that connects personal memory with history for each individual in the space. Basic movement ideas for *Körper* were thus developed by Sasha Waltz and the company in response to Libeskind's space as it confronted each body with German-Jewish history, before they started the final rehearsals at the Schaubühne.

Body Trilogy I: *Körper* (2000)

Research and inspiration for *Körper* initially derived from an interest Sasha Waltz took in the theme of "Being Human" – a project she collaborated on in preparation for the EXPO 2000 Hannover (Schlagenwerth,

2008, p. 60). While this project did not materialize in the end, Sasha Waltz pursued elements of the discussion into an in-depth research on the body in her choreographic work produced at the Schaubühne. *Körper* (2000) – the first part of the trilogy – investigated body-systems by taking a scientific–analytical approach towards the body – especially in those instances where the dancers are naked to avoid any eroticized or sexual connotation. Other themes of the choreography are "body and space" – in particular the focus on measuring the body to make space visible – as well as "body and medicine" to address recent developments in science and technology to stay young and fit. Lastly, the complex "body and history" emerged from her rehearsal process in the Jewish Museum (Schlagenwerth, 2008, p. 62). Body functions and anatomy fill the first half of the performance, when dancers crawl reminiscent of insects behind the large vertical glass vitrine, pull each other across the stage floor by the skin, paint organs for sale onto their lungs and heart ("hundred thousand Deutschmark") or spill water from a bottle between them to signify the amount of water stored by the living organism. The examination here relates to the discrepancy of the physical body as an object and the experiential body of the dancer as an individual person in society.

When the Portuguese dancer Claudia de Serpa Soares steps forward in a see-through red shirt-dress to announce "This is my body ..." pointing at her breasts for eyes and her front for her back, language is exposed as a misleading conveyor of truth. Costume designer Bernd Skodzig had worked with photo-cards of the dancers to tease out their individual corporeality and stage presence emphasizing physique and expression in the shape and material of the costumes he designed (see DVD "Körper", 2011). The choreography thus juxtaposes the neutral – naked – body as opposed to the expressive, social and personal body of the dancer. Themes from the rehearsal score for this section are "Eggs" – five-armed Takako Suzuki balancing three white eggs in the palm of one male and two female hands (with another two dancers hidden behind her); "Resistance" – starting as a trio dance between Juan Kruz Diaz de Garaio Esnaola, Joakim NaBi Olsson and Claudia de Serpa Soares before other company members join; "Skin" – company members dragging and pulling each other by the skin; "Transplantation and Operation", "Cleaning", "Measure", "Perfect Body", "Amok", "Nervous System", etc. The sequences are loosely held together underscored by the atmospheric acoustics by sound artist Hans Peter Kuhn. Often the

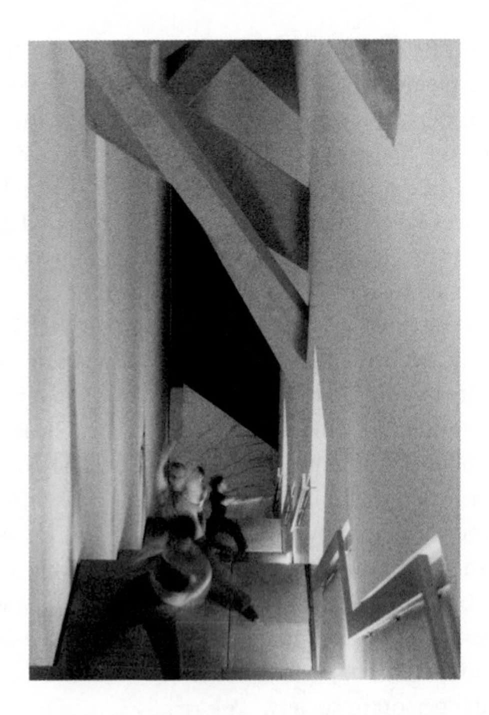

Dialoge '99/II **- Jüdisches Museum (1999) © Photo: Bernd Uhlig.**

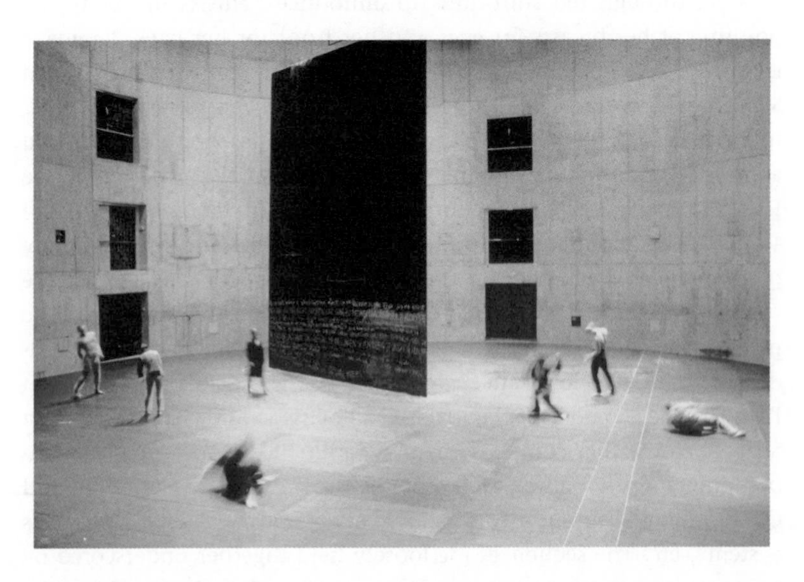

Körper **von Sasha Waltz / Hans Peter Kuhn (2000) © Photo: Bernd Uhlig.**

sound creates a metallic coldness that matches the vast empty space of the Schaubühne, a scratching, machine-like noise that de-humanizes some of the movements and coheres around the group as being pulled by some abstract, alienating, energetic force. In other instances, especially after the vertical black wall in the middle of the otherwise empty space has fallen down flat, the atmosphere changes at times introducing a more melancholy accordion-type tune for several duets and trios later on.

Body and deconstruction

Between the human and anti-human, Waltz's *Körper* interrogates the discursive formation of the body from a post-structuralist perspective of deconstruction in the wake of French philosopher Jacques Derrida (1930–2004). Derrida's two major works *Writing and Difference* (1978) and *Of Grammatology* (1976) critiqued Western logocentrism from the perspective of deferral by arguing that any linguistic meaning as the relationship between a sign and its object can never be fully determined or fixed. However, he was also critical and opposed to the phenomenological privileging of experience and presence as he believed those did strictly speaking not exist as they were always founded on our understanding of the past as we looked at with Merleau-Ponty in a previous chapter. Deconstruction is thus a philosophical method whereby the alleged truth of a written text, but also language and ultimately even subjective experience, are permanently questioned. For Derrida there is no substance, felt intuition or soul as a metaphysical concept to hold onto as human existence is endlessly caught up in the structuralist entanglement of interrelated but ultimately always withheld meanings.

Politically, this was an important strategy as it allowed for new identity positions to emerge throughout the 1970s and 1980s, however, ethically the void post-structuralist thinking produces at the heart of the meaning-making process is difficult if not impractical to live with. In that sense, Derrida's thought appears caught up in its own paradox, whereby human existence will always produce meanings, even if they are not founded on substance. A fact which he himself recognized and named as the "trace": the rupture of the void against metaphysics if you wish. This trace is also visible in Sasha Waltz's *Körper*, where language and costuming rub against the abstraction of the naked, dancing body. The post-structuralist perspective of deconstruction, however, stops at the limit of the physically palpable energetic core that constitutes the human body as an individual and in the group. As Australian dancer Grayson Milwood announces towards the end of the piece in a story he tells about his girlfriend "I wanted to show her everything about me that makes me different from everybody else" – difference and identity shine through the work as the two big topics of dance and theatre in the 1990s. While imagery of the Holocaust appears in abstraction – the measuring of bodies against the cold, concrete walls; naked bodies lying on top of each other, anonymized, lifeless – *Körper* never dwells on the illustrative but always keeps the necessary distance that the abstraction allows for. And yet, as the dancers fill the empty space, the invisible does become visible for the inner eye of the spectator as a felt emotional quality similar to the experience one gains when walking through Libeskind's axes underground the Jewish museum.

If Pina Bausch had already paved the ground for this uniquely West German genre of dance theatre after Laban, Wigman and Jooss in Wuppertal, Sasha Waltz and Guests redefined the image of Berlin after the Wall as a cosmopolitan European city. The company itself was formed around a group of international dancers born in the late 1960s to mid-1970s coming from Australia, Israel, Japan, Canada, Korea, Sweden, Lithuania, New Zealand, Portugal and Spain (see Stocker, 2003). The installation *Insideout* (2003) addressed questions of identity and globalization interrogating cultural theory ranging from Bourdieu to Sennett in the context of a group of young dancers from various national and cultural backgrounds working in Berlin. The individual body in Waltz's choreography is also always a group body forming the social organism. In confrontation with German history during the first decade after reunification, her international company set a model for a new Europe in the making. In this respect Waltz's location in Berlin appeared significant at a moment when reunification of East and West brought up questions of possible reconciliation with the wounds of the past towards further European integration creating the European Union under its current name with the establishing of the Maastricht Treaty in 1993. However, globalization, internationalization and the opening of the financial markets held its own challenges in store as we will see with some of the work we discuss in the next chapter.

Study Questions:

1. Judith Butler defines gender identity as "a stylized repetition of acts". Describe how the choreographers discussed in this chapter address the use of repetition as a choreographic tool. What are some of the political effects? Consider the influence on gay and women's rights for example.
2. Dance theatre does not introduce characters as we know them from realist stage convention or TV drama. What is the difference between movement and text? What are some of the strategies choreographers use in rehearsal?
3. To what extent does dance theatre reference everyday behaviour, how is it altered and what is your reaction as an audience member? Recall earlier definitions of Brecht's gestus, Grotowski's reference to the "social mask" or Bourdieu's "habitus".
4. Get together in groups of three and work on an abstraction of everyday movement, using primarily repetition and movement as your strategy. Think about the power dynamic in the group and how the repetition shifts your perception. Reflect upon the meaning of your sequence. How does it feel as opposed to what it looks like?
5. Develop the previous exercise introducing a textual element.

8 From Decolonization to Globalization

Discourses of Freedom and Emancipation in Wole Soyinka, Alvin Ailey, Bill T. Jones, Akram Khan and Sidi Larbi Cherkaoui

Postcolonial performance: Decolonizing Western theatre through dance

Cultural and postcolonial studies since the late 1970s until today are devoted to the study of the politics and cultural dynamic of the history of Western colonialism and the expanse of capitalism and mass media under globalization. Founded in the late 1950s into 1960s British-based cultural studies, represented by left-wing scholars such as Raymond Williams (1921–1988), Stuart Hall (1932–2014) and Paul Gilroy (*1956), started to examine popular culture and its impact on the political representation of the working classes as well as the African and South Asian diasporas in the work of the latter two. Paul Gilroy's influential *The Black Atlantic. Modernity and Double Consciousness* (1993) appeared at the high time of the cultural studies' movement in academia reflecting the important research of Birmingham's Centre for Contemporary Cultural Studies before it was forced to shut down by the conservative-leaning university administration in 2002. Gilroy drew attention to the impact of the slave trade on African diasporic culture that migrated across the Atlantic from the West African coast into the Caribbean islands, South and North America. Cultural studies set out to examine the politics of class, race and gender as they intersected with the discourses of modernity and nationalism. Gilroy's study pointed out how cultural nationalism was often defined via an ethnic essentialism which in the British case, for example, refers to cultural signifiers of Englishness. While the nation was traditionally considered an "ethnically homogenous object" (Gilroy, 1993, p. 3), the histories of European colonial imperialism and reversed migration into cities like London, Paris and Brussels since the 1950s complicated such ethnocentric narratives. As Gilroy points out,

> These modes of subjectivity and identification acquire a renewed political charge in the post-imperial history that saw black settlers from Britain's colonies take up their citizenship rights as subjects in the United Kingdom. The entry of blacks into national life was itself a powerful factor contributing to the circumstances in which the formation of both cultural studies and new Left politics became possible. It indexes the profound transformations of British social and cultural life in the 1950s and stands, again usually unacknowledged, at the heart of laments for a more human scale of social living that seemed no longer practicable after the 1939–45 war. (1993, p. 10)

Such transformation of the social life occurred across different migratory communities in Britain including African and African-Caribbean as well as South Asian migrants and their families. Gilroy emphasized the importance of cultural expression as a binding force in the diaspora with particular focus on music which, however, can easily be adapted for dance as these are usually interdependent in Africanist and South Asian performance cultures.

Postcolonial studies, on the other hand, emerged initially from the critical reception of French post-structuralism in US academia. Edward Said (1935–2003) is perhaps to be considered the discipline's founding figure with his key publications *Orientalism* (1978) and *Culture and Imperialism* (1994). He critiqued the Western colonial bias that has shaped literature and media representation of the so-called "others" in the former colonies. Influenced by Michel Foucault's writings on discourse analysis, Said's project set out to deconstruct Western stereotypical views and strategies of othering in literature, arts and media. A postcolonial perspective hence investigates constructions of identity as other. If we think about the set-up of the colonial situation, then colonialism made a distinction between colonizers (mostly European) and colonized (mostly non-European). Such a distinction is powerful because it allows political elites to justify the oppression of other people by stereotyping and discriminating against them on the ground of their difference in appearance, social status or gender. This mode of thinking goes back to the eighteenth-century German philosopher Friedrich Hegel (1770–1831) who in his *Phenomenology of Mind* declared that we each develop our own notion of self in relation to another. Important for his argument is the fact that we mostly seek recognition or identification from or with other people in terms of developing a stable self-confidence. This, however, is only possible if we are recognized as equal to our peers. If, on the other hand, such equality or similarity is not given or denied, we psychologically experience insecurity of self and may even start to develop complexes and anxieties. Such differences manifest themselves in the face of an encounter between different ethnicities and cultures, different class systems and also with gender.

In the wake of Said's pioneering efforts, Gayatri Spivak (*1942) and Homi K. Bhabha (*1949) further defined the field of postcolonialism as a critical theory for the analysis of literature and culture. Spivak's work in so-called subaltern studies critically examined the role of women as most disenfranchised by the colonialist legacy. In her seminal essay "Can the Subaltern Speak?" (1985), she questioned whether the formerly colonized have a voice to speak for themselves or whether they are condemned to be forever represented through the agents of colonial power. Homi K. Bhabha's groundbreaking *The Location of Culture* (1994) coined two other key terms in postcolonial studies, namely, "mimicry" and "hybridity" to describe the multicultural landscape after the Second World War. A key figure for Bhabha to develop mimicry and hybridity as critical concepts was Frantz Fanon (1925–1961). Fanon was a psychiatrist from Martinique who in his seminal works *Black Skin, White Masks* (1952) and *The Wretched of the Earth* (1961) critiqued the issue of colonial oppression in the French Antilles. His main discovery was that he found a prevalent psychopathology with his African Caribbean patients who felt deprived of their self-confidence based on their colour of skin, especially when confronted with the discrimination by white people as the former colonizers. The title *Black Skin, White Masks* referred to the irony of a colonialist politics – particularly under French rule – which considered the colony as a part of France in terms of education and administration, yet denied full acceptance of the colonized as French on the grounds of skin colour and a nineteenth-century rhetoric of racial segregation. Fanon was the first postcolonial scholar to describe the vicious circle of racial oppression by demonstrating long-lasting psychological trauma caused by a colonialist politics that codified black skin to represent the colonized or oppressed, while white skin was cast as the leading discourse of power and privilege. His acute analysis dismantled how colonial discourse operates by manipulating language and images to create derogatory and stereotypical attitudes towards black people. And yet, as we read Fanon, we also start to see through this discriminatory mechanism so that racism as a discourse of representation can slowly be undermined.

What differentiates Bhabha's approach from Fanon and Hegel is that he locates identity in-between sameness and difference rather than determined as the one or the other. For Bhabha the relationship between self and other is thus a little more complex in that he points to the fact that identity construction is an ongoing and open process. In his writings he calls this the ambivalence of the colonial encounter and suggests that stereotypes are never fixed. Bhabha refers back to Fanon's example of a prevalent white racism, yet questions its power. Stereotypes, so Bhabha argues, may indeed lead to an inferiority complex, however – unlike Fanon – Bhabha does not believe that the discourse must necessarily stay fixed at that level. Instead he stresses that colonialism is no one-way street, and that white self-perception was as much changed in the colonial encounter. He therefore proposes the term "mimicry" to refer to an imitative behaviour whereby blacks try to become white or whites try to become black (something we may see more often today, in hip-hop culture for example) in order to creatively subvert the discriminating stereotype.

Note that Bhabha's concept of mimicry as a mode of defence and camouflage is very theatrical – there is the word mimesis or imitation part of its etymological root – as is also Fanon's image of the mask in his writing. Performances are considered postcolonial, when they demonstrate either an anti-imperialistic agenda or a political subversive strategy in terms of reversing the power dynamic between colonizers and colonized. By taking this perspective we can interpret theatre and dance as a direct response to colonialism and analyse how they contribute to the rewriting of history. Postcolonial performances may then serve indigenous communities to regenerate their cultural heritage and find new pride in sharing cultural traditions to nurture self-esteem (see Gilbert and Tompkins, 1996; Balme, 1999). Syncretic theatre is another term we may use, and it differs slightly in terms of referring rather more to the aesthetic implications of postcolonial theatre than its political effects (see Balme, 1999). When we speak of syncretic theatre, we look at cultural fusion, the use of ritual, oral traditions, dance and carnival from diverse backgrounds and how they shift our understanding of the body in Western theatre and performance.

The approaches of cultural and postcolonial studies share in common the examination of culture from its broadest angle including literary texts, film and TV, radio as well as music and dance in order to analyse their formative dimension as a political strategy of representation. Gilroy's *Black Atlantic* claimed African diasporic music as a powerful articulation of pan-African political solidarity across national divides, whereas Bhabha's concept of hybridity argued for the creative-subversive politics of cultural mimicry which – as the product of many cultures – will always produce something new even if necessarily speaking strategically from within the discourse of power. Post-structuralist thought is important in this context, because both Foucault's discourse analysis as well as Derrida's notion of differance state that cultural identities are not stable, but depend on the historical context and prevalent power dynamic in any given society at a time. Racism and misogyny are thus enabled by the performative use of language and culture that privileges lighter phenotypes and men over women when it comes to voting rights, salaries and other areas of possible discrimination. Post-structuralism argues that such discrimination can be subverted, because it is performative meaning that it is based on our socially agreed use of language. Post-structuralist deconstruction highlights the gap whereby meaning is never absolute but deferred and open to change. Language is only truthful by cultural agreement so that we can change the meaning and connotations of words over time. There is a distinct political edge to postcolonial analysis in that it seeks to activate its audiences whether they are readers or theatre-goers as well as to give agency, meaning a voice, to the oppressed. And finally, it is concerned with the question of cultural identity and self-definition in an increasingly complex and diverse world, mainly addressing the issue of the status of human rights and dignity from a cross-cultural perspective. In the following analysis of dance in Western theatre we will see how dance performance enabled such deconstruction of colonial stereotype as we move historically from decolonization towards globalization during the second half of the twentieth century into the twenty-first century.

Decolonizing drama: Wole Soyinka's *Death and the King's Horseman*

Wole Soyinka was born in Aké, near Abeokuta in Western Nigeria. His father was a distinguished teacher and his mother a trader deeply involved in the cultural and social life of her community. Soyinka was educated at the University College of Ibadan, where he obtained a scholarship for further study abroad. He chose the University of Leeds, where he received a degree in English literature in 1957. At Leeds he studied with G. Wilson Knight, a renowned Shakespeare scholar of the time and the critic Arnold Kettle, both of whom he later acknowledged as strong influences on his own writing. Soyinka went on to the Royal Court Theatre and joined a group of emerging playwrights under George Devine. In 1960 he returned to Nigeria on a Rockefeller Fellowship to study African theatre traditions, he also started teaching drama and literature at Ibadan and founded his own theatre troupe. From early on Soyinka has been involved in writing and political activity which instantly got him into conflict with the local political authorities. Starting with a first period of police detention, when in 1965 he was accused of being a masked gunman who had forced the local Ibadan broadcasting station to replace a tape by the then Premier of the region with one protesting against him. However, at the time, the judges cast the benefit of the doubt and released Soyinka from prison. When in 1967 the Nigerian Civil War – also known as the Nigerian-Biafran War – broke out, Soyinka was involved in peacemaking efforts to appeal for a ceasefire between the factions at war. He travelled to Biafra, the secessionist enclave, and was arrested for allegedly conspiring with the rebels there. For twenty-seven months he was held as a political prisoner, twenty-two of those in solitary confinement. Soyinka is not only recognized as an accomplished playwright, but he also wrote several autobiographical accounts as well as novels and poetry. In 1986 he was the first writer of African descent to be awarded the Nobel Prize for Literature.

Death and the King's Horseman is perhaps Soyinka's most studied play. The plot was drawn from real events that took place in Nigeria in 1946 and can still be found in the archives of the British colonial administration today. As Soyinka mentions in the "Author's Note" to the play, that year "the lives of Elesin (Olori Elesin), his son, and the Colonial District Officer intertwined" in a way that brings about the tragedy of the play

(1993, p. 3). What are these events? The King of Oyo, the ancient city of the Yoruba, has died and therefore his horseman, Elesin, is expected to follow him in death according to the Yoruba belief system. The play opens as the preparations for this ritual death or suicide begin to unfold, and we get a sense of the dancing and drumming this involves as well as through the imagery and poetic language used in the opening scene between Elesin and the Praise-Singer as well as the preparations by Iyaloja, his wife, and the market women. At the same time the British colonial officer, Pilkings, is expecting the visit of the British royalty and he is afraid of an insurrection caused by the events surrounding Elesin's death.

The tragedy thus unfolds from two sources: (a) a misunderstanding of cultural traditions, but also, and this is Soyinka's favoured interpretation, (b) the metaphysical dilemma which Elesin finds himself in, derived from the complexity of the Yoruba world view and cosmological beliefs. As Soyinka suggests,

> The confrontation in the play is largely metaphysical, contained in the human vehicle which is Elesin and the universe of the Yoruba mind – the world of the living, the dead and the unborn, and the numinous passage which links all: transition. Death and the King's Horseman can be fully realised only through an evocation of music from the abyss of transition (1993, p. 4).

Here Soyinka's dramaturgy brings together kinaesthetic memory derived from the Yoruba in Nigeria with Western models of drama and tragedy. While a British audience will be able to easily discern the Western dramatic form of scenic divisions and dialogue, a Nigerian public will more easily relate to the autochthonous performance elements of dance and singing included in the stage directions for the production of the play and in particular its challenging opening scene written as an homage to Yoruba ritual and poetry.

Dance, drama and ritual: Tragedy and Yoruba cosmology in the play

The Yoruba in Nigeria inhabit a complex belief system, where the living people share intimate relationships with their ancestors, deities and the unborn. Their perception of time and history transcends the individual's life cycle and is intimately held within the community's ritual performances of cultural memory. It is important to realize this connection for our analysis of dance and embodiment in *Death and the King's Horseman*, because Yoruba cosmology is at the heart of Elesin's tragic fate. The opening scene evokes the poetic style and complex imagery of Yoruba song and myth building up to the incantation of the "Not-I Bird" dance ritual (Soyinka, 1993, p. 9). As the King's horseman, Elesin starts out as a greatly admired man in the community. Such admiration, however, also comes with very specific culturally coded expectations and responsibilities towards the community. For example, Iyaloja and the women expect him to be prepared and ready to follow his King into death. However, as we can see reflected in the song and dance of the "Not-I Bird" Elesin's departure from life is not entirely easy on him, and we get a sense of regret for life as he seeks to have another wife just before he leaves at the end of the first scene.

"Not-I", in the opening song and dance, refers to the various instances of people enjoying life and fleeing from death and the setting up of Elesin as the brave man who will not falter and follow his king into death performing a ritualized suicide as the Yoruba custom demands (Soyinka, 1993, pp. 10–17). While the women of the market led by Iyaloja prepare to dress him in finest robes, his attention is caught by a young woman distracting his mind from his ritualistic purpose (Soyinka, 1993, pp. 17–18). Even though the young woman is to be married to his own son, Elesin demands to be wed to her on the same night as to mark his passage by a sexual union that may bring forth new life (Soyinka, 1993, p. 21). Since the ritual has already begun, the women led by Iyaloja dare not deny his wish, although it remains unclear whether Elesin speaks ancestral wisdom indeed or merely seeks to gratify his sexual pleasure (Soyinka, 1993, p. 22).

Dance during this scene symbolizes the transition between the world of the living and the world of the ancestors. The drumming and dancing evoke Ashé a differently charged energy that describes the life force in Yoruba mythology. Elesin's ritualistic dance creates a different dimensionality, already half-removed from the world of the living and entering the ancestral realm. His words appear to be taken for the words of the ancestors, although we also sense some doubt in Iyaloja's replies. This hints at the interference and rupture already taking place within the Yoruba community as a consequence of the colonial contact. The fact that the play was written in English and introduces doubt and debate also questions the effective continuity of tradition and custom as they are presented through the dramatist's lens. Nonetheless, Soyinka's mastery consists precisely in writing the play such that a culturally sensitive production will make this conflict between language, rational thought and the wisdom embodied in cultural memory and dance viscerally palpable on stage.

The next important ritualistic aspect of the play is introduced in the second scene with the appearance of the Egungun masks (Soyinka, 1993, pp. 24–36). Egungun masks are not costumes in the Western sense, but rather sacred manifestations of the ancestors. These masks are kept in secret and will only be worn by selected men of the Yoruba community on occasion of specific ceremonies. An Egungun mask covers the entire body of the performer, and accompanied by specific drum rhythms and dancing, they bring the ancestor back into the world. Margaret Thompson Drewal describes the impact of the dancing Egungun mask as such:

> The masks manifest the spirits of ancestors. As such, the masks are nonfigurative. Their synthesis of costume and movement totally transforms the human body into an abstract kinetic sculpture. These masks allude to the nonhuman qualities of spirits. In their movement, the dancers strive for a more thoroughly integrated dancing image in which legs and arms are often imperceptible. To communicate their liminal states, Egungun use altered voice qualities, wear amorphous cloth forms conceived and sewn in ways to obscure or to alter human features, carry dangerous medicines on their person that prohibit outsiders and uninitiated from touching them out of fear of sickness or death, and perform highly stylized dances. (2003, p. 124)

If we understand the impact of the Egungun mask and dance in Yoruba culture, we can see how Pilkings and his wife offend their servants by dishonouring their spiritual power. The use of the Egungun also highlights that a Western audience will probably have a very different understanding of the scene by mistaking it for a carnival costume compared to Nigerian audiences who are familiar with the sacred tradition in the Yoruba context.

Soyinka's use of drumming and dancing throughout the play serves as a dramaturgical device in the play to highlight the rising tension. Notice how drumming in scene two creates an unsettling atmosphere throughout and how the alleged noise cannot be deciphered clearly as it announces the wedding and the death of the King's horseman at the same time (Soyinka, 1993, p. 32). Yoruba drums are talking drums, which means that their pitching functions in a structure very similar to Yoruba language and has been used as a means of communication and signalling. As Peter Badejo explains their function upon a visit of the Oyo Palace in ancient Yoruba land for Rufus Norris's 2009 production at the National Theatre in London:

> Besides the drums' ability to make people dance and understand their language, the "dùndún" is used to communicate. For example when Rufus [Norris, the director], Javier [de Frutos, the choreographer] and I went to the Oyo Palace, the drummers were welcoming us in but, at the same time, they were telling the chiefs inside the Palace what kind of people they should be expecting. If they didn't want to see us, by the time we got to the next gate they could say they're not at home. It's a means of communication not unlike the traditional telephone! (NT Program 2009)

Apart from the ritualistic elements in the play, Soyinka also picks up Bhabha's concept of mimicry in a character such as Amusa who is ridiculed as a "white man's eunuch" (1993, p. 36) by the market women in scene three. Soyinka uses language to portray the arrogance of the colonial administration in a satirical mock-imitation that reverses the colonial stereotype (1993, pp. 40–42).

Dance features as a central key to cultural memory, ritual and embodiment among the Yoruba and allows Soyinka's dramaturgy for the play to reverse our perspective on Western cultural values. The 2009 production at the National Theatre capitalized on the choreographic elements by staging the play in the semi-round and also introducing the idea of a masque for the carnival scene that played with Western court dance as opposed to the African ritual dance being performed in the background. An all-black cast wore white masks to reverse some of the colonial politics as well. By introducing a character such as Olunde, Elesin's son, Soyinka set the incidents a couple of years earlier than they actually happened as to have Elesin's ritual suicide coincide with the Second World War in Europe. Through Olunde the play addresses the question of cultural relativism by posing several important questions towards the end of the play. For example, what do we consider more

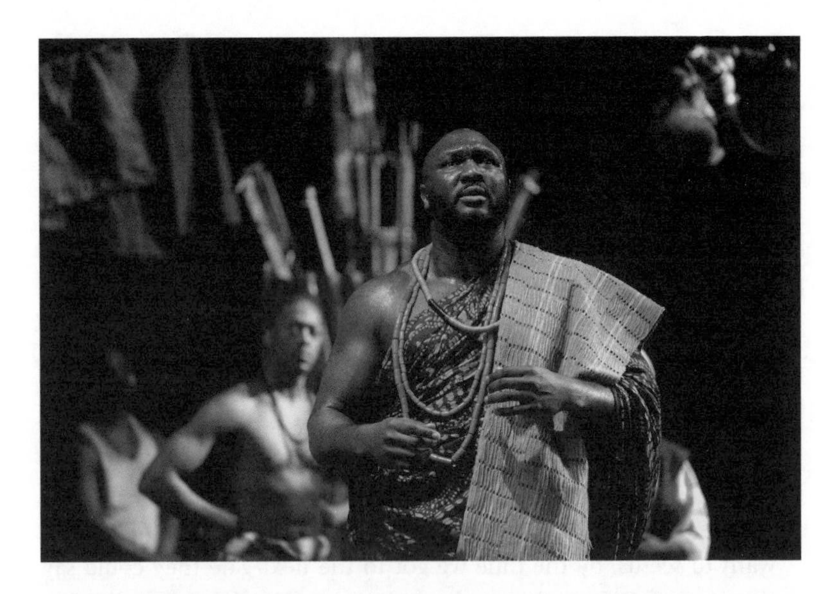

Nonso Anozie as Elesin, Horseman of the King in *Death and the King's Horseman*, directed by Rufus Norris at NT 2009 © Robbie Jack.

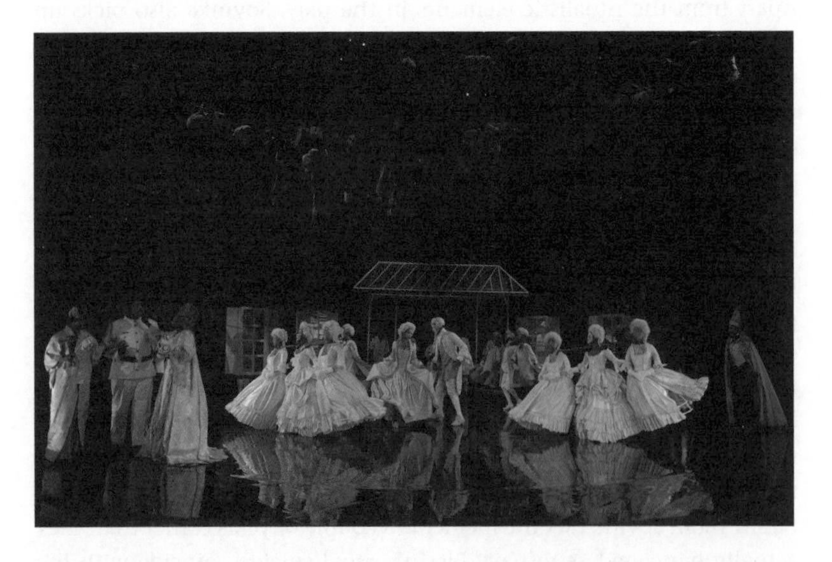

***Death and the King's Horseman*, directed by Rufus Norris at NT 2009 © Robbie Jack.**

barbaric: An individual who dies because of religious belief in his death as a guarantee for the life of the community or millions of people dead in a war in Europe? These are difficult questions raised by the play, and Soyinka does not give us any easy answers to them. However, if we consider the significance of ritual dance among the Yoruba, it seems that the ritual suicide was a transition into life (= Ashé) rather than death in the Western sense. Fundamentally, dance signifies yet again a different temporality and ethics closely tied to performative practice and cultural identity.

Black Atlantic performance: The modern dance theatre of Alvin Ailey (1931–1989)

The modern dance theatre of Alvin Ailey emerged alongside the dance and theatre works created by Martha Graham, Merce Cunningham, the Living Theatre and Yvonne Rainer. During those turbulent years of political change between 1954 and 1968, African Americans were fighting for civil rights, and dance played no small part in supporting the struggle. American modern dance was influenced by the impact of African diasporic cultures since its very beginnings. The Atlantic slave trade lasted from the fifteenth into the nineteenth centuries, and it is estimated that 12 to 20 million African people fell victim to its forced deportations (see Guérivière, 2004, Soyinka, 1999). Ever since African Americans first arrived on the American continent, their cultural traditions have shaped American culture as a unique blend of different aesthetic principles and creative ideas. The history of slavery and racial segregation in the United States forms the background to the political relevance of Alvin Ailey's work at the time, but it also points towards an understanding of the importance of dance and embodiment when it comes to cultural memory and survival (see DeFrantz, 2004).

Underlying African diasporic dance forms, one finds a set of commonalities that align Africanist movement aesthetics across different African performance traditions past and present (see Sloat, 2002). Art historian Robert Farris Thompson was among the first to filter the following shared characteristics of African American sculptural forms: ephebism (= "a youthful quality"), balance, social, circular and call-and-response (Thompson, 1974, p. 27). In his wake, dance scholars Kariamu Welsh Asante (see 2001, 1996) and Brenda Dixon Gottschild (see 2003, 1998) have also found these to be represented in Africanist dance forms. Welsh-Asante's model outlines the following elements of Africanist dance aesthetics: polyrhythms and polycentrism, dimensionality of the spirit pantheon and cosmological context, curvilinear shapes and forms, epic memory, repetition, and an overarching sensibility of holism (2001, pp. 144–151). Retentions of Africanist movement principles in modern dance form part of what I have elsewhere referred to as "kinaesthetic memory" based on Joseph Roach's analysis of cultural surrogation in Circum-Atlantic performances (Roach, 1996). Kinaesthetic memory thus speaks to the complex creative transformation that takes place in choreographic processes that merge Africanist movement retentions with Western European dance vocabularies in the context of postcolonial nation building such as in the case of The National Dance Theatre Company of Jamaica (Sörgel, 2007, pp. 96–98). Africanist retentions in the Caribbean, South America and the United States form part of an embodied cultural memory that has shaped cultural identity over generations and as such testifies to the survival of cultural heritage beyond the trauma of the Middle Passage. Kinaesthetic memory thus links the African diaspora across different continents and establishes affiliations that are transnational. In this respect the dance works in this chapter exemplify the importance of dance for cultural heritage in a postcolonial and diasporic context. As we now move from decolonization towards globalization in the second half of the twentieth century, we will see how dance enables powerful cultural alliances across different countries and continents.

Revelations (1960)

Alvin Ailey's *Revelations* (1960) is undoubtedly his signature piece and one of the classics of modern dance history. Based on Ailey's memories of Texas, where he grew up in an environment of black Christianity, the choreography evokes many instances of religious syncretism between African and Christian belief systems, kinaesthetic memory and spirituality expressed in song and dance. The choreography is divided into three sections encompassing a suite of three gospel songs for sections one, two and four for the final one. In the beginning, the stage is dark and then the lights go up on a choric body raising hands up in what appear to be signature moves of the modern dance lineage derived from Lester Horton, Martha Graham and Doris Humphrey (DeFrantz, 2004, p. 15). "I've been buked" is the first song of the section called "Pilgrim of Sorrow", to then lead into a dance duet to "Didn't my Lord deliver Daniel" and the solo "Fix me Jesus" commemorating the pain of slavery that marks African American experience as the traumatic struggle towards freedom (DeFrantz, 2004, pp. 5–9). Spirituals in the African American tradition are songs of freedom and embody the deliverance from slavery as expressed by the upward, vertical orientation of the lifted palms touching an imagined heaven, "breathing" through the vocal accompaniment (DeFrantz, 2004, p. 14).

The next section "Take me to the Water" speaks of kinaesthetic memory and survival of African dance forms and religious beliefs that aligned Christian river baptism with the Yoruba cosmological beliefs in Oshun as evoked by the white costumes and rippling shoulder movements of damaballah the serpent energy that mobilizes the spine in Haitian Vodoun as was filmed and documented by Maya Deren's early experimental documentary *Divine Horsemen* as well as taught by Katherine Dunham based on her research in the Caribbean. The songs "Processional", "Wading in the Water" and "I want to be ready" speak of the healing powers associated with the memory of the dance forms that survived the Middle Passage and sustained African cultural survival and community in the diaspora. Finally, therefore, the third section "Move, Members, Move" transcends sorrow and pain into spiritual deliverance that overcomes the alienation of separation and trauma. As Thomas DeFrantz's seminal study on the company commented on this transition of styles:

> Here, dancers rarely look toward each other or the audience. They are sorrowful, beaten, without individual agency. The modern enervates them, saps their bodies of dynamic potential. Significantly, as *Revelations* becomes more jubilant, its movements migrate from (white) modernist abstraction to (black) vernacular dance structures. The dancers escape the dead confines of abstract dance that expresses inner turmoil to inhabit the living representation of people dancing for and with each other. (2004, p. 22)

In DeFrantz's reading, the first section pays homage to dance modernism as an abstract form of dance primarily serving the expression of white female subjectivity as we discussed with Martha Graham before (2004, p. 21). While African American dancers such as Pearl Primus (1919–1994) and Katherine Dunham (1909–2006), as well as Asadata Dafora (1890–1965) had created solo works which explored West African and African Caribbean dance forms before, Alvin Ailey was the first to successfully install his own company trained in diverse modern dance techniques and ballet. Black dancers became visible on the US concert stage by adopting a style of dance white American audiences were already familiar with, yet by incorporating black vernacular dances and cultural memories, they were able to speak to their own community in a more direct way and express themselves gaining respect and public recognition through the international acclaim of their art work (DeFrantz, 2004, p. 21). Alvin Ailey's American Dance Theatre thus played an important part ushering into the Civil Rights Movement alongside the non-violent protests spearheaded by Martin Luther King at the time.

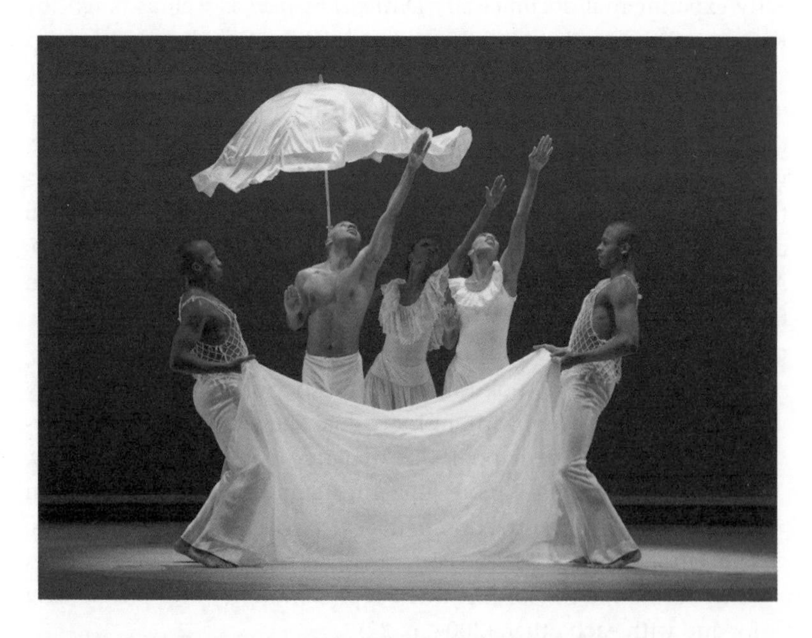

Alvin Ailey American Dance Theatre in *Revelations*, dancers: Christopher Jackson, Matthew Rushing, Renee Robinson, Constance Stamatiou & Yannick Lebrun © Nan Melville.

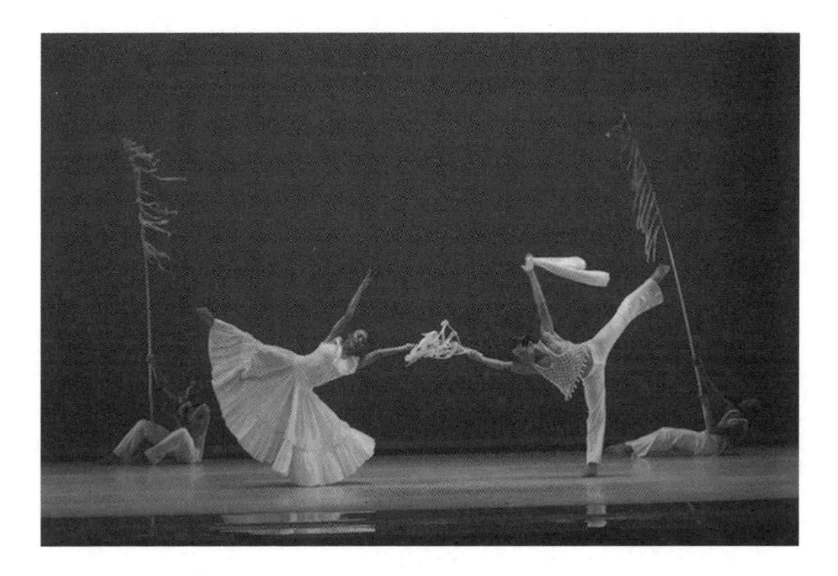

Alvin Ailey American Dance Theatre in *Revelations* © Nan Melville.

Black Atlantic performance post Civil Rights: Bill T. Jones and Arnie Zane Dance Company

Last Supper at Uncle Tom's Cabin/ The Promised Land (1990) contextualizes Bill T. Jones's work of the 1990s as deeply involved in American identity politics. Bill T. Jones (*1952) and Arnie Zane (1948–1988) emerged out of the 1970s postmodern dance movement and their interracial dance, created together with Lois Welk for their first company called American Dance Asylum, spurred a new cultural politics debating social values after civil rights. Their dance was grounded in contact improvisation, the free method of movement vocabulary evolved by Steve Paxton, and often highly energetic blending of spoken and dance sections with striking visual media effects, such as in *Everybody Works/All Beasts Count* (1975) and *At The Crux* (1976). Improvising, the two dancers dovetailed their later duets *Blauvelt Mountain* (1980) and *Valley Cottage* (1980) with highly autobiographical onstage dialogues – a technique that you will still find present in the company's training as evidenced in the documentary on the making of *Last Supper at Uncle Tom's Cabin* (2004).

Jones and Zane were partners in life and art, and their homosexual relationship raised a cultural debate on identity politics in the Jewish and African American community during the 1980s. Jones and Zane emphasized and explored their cultural differences but also explored cross-gender casting with company members coming from different cultural backgrounds. Their choreography sought to break away from racial segregation by promoting identity and difference in their work. Zane died prematurely of HIV in the 1980s causing Bill T. Jones to publicly announce his own HIV positive status at the time. Dance and survival evolved as themes which the dance company addressed to cope with the mourning and loss of a generation traumatized by the HIV in highly acclaimed works such as *D Man in the Waters* (1989) and *Still/Here* (1994). Throughout his dance career Bill T. Jones has worked across genres and styles by blending elements from theatre, film, classical music and jazz in his choreographic work as also most recently in the Broadway musical hit *Fela!* (2008) on the Nigerian Afrobeats musician Fela Kuti.

Last Supper at Uncle Tom's Cabin/The Promised Land (1990): Choreographic sources

Bill T. Jones's approach to choreography often starts from autobiographical soul-searching to question myths of American culture and identity. His choreographic oeuvre explores themes of racism, sexuality and faith with roots in his own life experience as a gay African American dancer. Together with his dance company he looks at multicultural America and its diversity built on the promise of the French Revolution and enlightenment values of life, liberty and the pursuit of happiness. For many people America has symbolized this haven of democracy, but at the same time the country's history of early settlement, colonization and slavery has scarred this promise of equality and egalitarianism. For African Americans, in particular, slavery and the struggle for civil rights have become landmarks of their emancipation struggle, self-definition and identification. As Bill T. Jones comments in the documentary: "This dance is a political poster (on the surface), but it is also about the people who are performing it" (2004).

The choreography investigates American democracy through the critical investigation of American myths on "race" and "motherhood" as embodied in the image of "Uncle Tom" and "Eliza" in Acts I and II of the dance epic. If you watch the excerpt of Act I "The Cabin", you will notice how Jones deconstructs the stereotypical myth of "Uncle Tom" as a "submissive, stoic and selfless" individual as characterized in Harriet Beecher Stowes's nineteenth-century sentimental novel and its influence on film that historian Donald Bogle refers to below:

> Always as toms are chased, harassed, hounded, flogged, enslaved, and insulted, they keep the faith, never turn against their white massas, and remain hearty, submissive, stoic, generous, selfless, and oh-so-very kind. Thus they endear themselves to white audiences and emerge as heroes of sorts. (1997, pp. 5–6)

In Act II Bill T. Jones picks up on the novel's character of Eliza, a mulatto slave woman who escapes from her mistress's house, because her slave master has sold her child to slave traders. Chapter 7 of the novel depicts "Eliza's dramatic" escape as she elopes from her brutal pursuers over the icy surface of a river. It is one of the early dramatic highpoints of the novel's naturalist plot as she is close to death, risking her life to save her child. The strength and bravery of motherhood is celebrated in this tragic heroine of nineteenth-century sentimentalism, which makes us identify with her and feel pity for her. While this is a somewhat limiting image of womanhood solely defined by her motherly feelings, it is at the same time employed as a powerful strategy to redefine the white gaze and imaginary on the inhumanity of slavery at the time. However, in his contemporary re-writing of this myth Bill T. Jones splits this character into three: performed by a light-skinned African American, a white woman and an African American dancer in drag. As a choreographer he thus deconstructs gender roles and racial stereotypes at the same time.

The "Promised Land Tour" took the choreography to several states in the United States and raised several controversies and social debates for its exploration of racism, sexuality, and faith. The choreography, Bill T. Jones has argued, explores these differences in order to work through them in the performance and arrive at another place of mutual tolerance and love. When the performers undress in the final scene, their naked bodies express this striving for commonality and the recognition and acceptance of these differences. As Bill T. Jones's says, "Every possible body should be there" (2004), and nakedness for him becomes an articulation of faith in this promise of human equality, where the performance crosses the border from art to life. Hutera summarizes the impact of this scene as follows:

> Combining the sweep of opera with the impact of political statement, the show presented images of power, struggle, sacrifice, humiliation, and oppression. By the finale, however, the fury and desperation fuelling the whole piece were set aside and overcome, as a swarm of dancers of all shapes and sizes filled and filed back and forth across the stage, united by their complete or (in some performances) partial nudity. (Hutera, 1999, p. 123)

Bill T. Jones's *Last Supper at Uncle Tom's Cabin/The Promised Land* presented a celebration of diversity and multiculturalism during the mid-1990s. In many ways, it represented a hopeful moment when civil rights had been accomplished for a large majority of US society. Choreographically, the work brought together narrative structures based in Alvin Ailey's tradition of dance theatre with a critical sensibility closer to postmodern dance and contact improvisation. At the same time, we also see how strategies of collaboration between the choreographer and his dancers allow for a more democratic creative process that integrates the embodied knowledge each performer brings to the stage as an individual.

Globalizing dance theatre: Akram Khan (*1974) and Sidi Larbi Cherkaoui (*1976)

Akram Khan and Sidi Larbi Cherkaoui are both contemporary dance choreographers who incorporate a diverse range of dance training in their creative process. Both dancers share a migratory background and interest in contemporary British and Flemish dance and dance theatre. In Khan's case via his education at De Montfort University as well as a period of working with Anne Teresa De Keersmaeker's Brussels-based X-Group project, and in Cherkaoui's career through his engagement with Les Ballets C de la B. However, both artists are also self-trained in the sense that they have made their own post-migrant autobiography part and parcel of their dance. Thus Khan was trained in classical Kathak since the age of seven under his teacher Sri Pratap Pwar, but he also toured with Peter Brook's *Mahabharata* at age thirteen for three years. Khan's parents moved from Bangladesh to London in the 1970s, and thus Khan's early training in Indian classical dance was influenced by his mother (Seibert, 2006, p. 17). At age seven, Khan enrolled in

Sri Pratap Pawar's Kathak School. Sri Pratap Pawar had been a disciple of Birju Maharaj and became Khan's guru for the next ten years.

To begin Kathak, the study of the music comes first, and it is perhaps here that the foundation for Khan's later choreographic work was laid, since his mind appears to continuously count according to Kathak's rhythmic patterns juxtaposing high-speed movement with abrupt moments of stillness. The musical pattern in Kathak is set, and yet because of that disciplined routine it allows then for endless variation and improvisation to occur in the rapport between dancer and master drummer (Seibert, 2006, p. 17). Khan enrolled at the Northern School of Contemporary Dance, which caused several "confusions" as Khan himself referred to this change in his Kathak trained body. While critics and dance scholarship appear divided over whether such confusion is desirable, there is a common denominator to claim such "liminal hybridity" (Mitra, 2009, p. 32) as an expression of contemporary British Asian identity in dance (see also Burt, 2004; Sanders, 2007; Mitra, 2015). Apart from the cultural reading, however, Khan's dance aesthetic also embodies an organic exploration of Kathak itself via contemporary dance methods. As Seibert describes this process:

> His guru had given him a discipline; his university studies had given him the freedom to question it. And the problem wasn't only mental. His body – that repository of tradition – was also confused; it didn't move like the bodies of the other dancers because it knew different things. Khan decided to listen to it, and in a series of solos he began to develop that rarest of things in dance: a new language, a new way of moving, clarity out of chaos. (2006, p. 17)

Such clarity, however, only emerges from a body in tune with the changing internal and external impulses. In a way, the vocabulary needs to sink in with the dancer's own personality responding to "internal, somatic sources" so that it becomes a truthful articulation rather than mere imitation of formal aspects (see Burt, 2004). Because Akram Khan is as much of a contemporary British citizen as he is a classically trained Kathak dancer, this exploration began to make new sense and speak of his own development in an adequate dance vocabulary and choreographic style.

Since 2000, Khan is the artistic director of his own company which he co-founded with Farooq Chaudry. Looking back, Khan acknowledges the role collaboration has played for him to develop his specific aesthetic and approach towards choreography. He believes that each work is not only influenced by the creativity of his many collaborators but also mirroring the explosion of media technology since the turn of the century (Khan, 2011). The company's founding ethos hence evolved from the idea of creating a "we" from as diverse sources as possible. Khan explains,

> To us, "We" in a collaborative sense means a sort of neutral space, where no "ONE" person leads, where no map is preconceived, in order to take a journey together. Farooq and I embraced the belief that, in order for us to grow, to learn to discover, we had to break limits, we had to break fixed patterns, to break set rituals that were given or passed down, and so we quickly realized that to cross any boundaries was another means to excuse for learning and discovering. (2011)

Such creative exploration of cultural and artistic boundaries undermines easy definitions of style marketing Khan's work as either contemporary or classical. However, what is really at stake for Khan is not so much an aesthetic quest, but rather seeking to investigate dance's potential to engage dancers and audiences in debates over values and moral standards involved in collaboration. Khan's collaborative performance ethic also influences the way he casts dancers for the company as well as how he trains them.

Sidi Larbi Cherkaoui and Akram Khan share a concern for the themes of "equality between individuals, cultures, languages and means of expression" (Cherkaoui, 2008, p. 12). Born in Antwerp, Cherkaoui grew up as the son of a Moroccan immigrant worker and started dancing in TV shows at the age of fourteen. Without any formal training, Cherkaoui's movement vocabulary derived from astute observation and mirroring of particular dance styles at first, while always integrating them into his own way of moving and thereby understanding the world. The TV shows brought him together with other dancers who recommended that he should take further training, and Cherkaoui enrolled in a higher school for dance in Antwerp where he was introduced to modern dance based on techniques such as Graham and Limón. In 1995 Cherkaoui met Alain Platel who organized a contest for "Best Belgian dancer" in Ghent that year with Wim van de Keybus as well as members of Anne Teresa De Keersmaeker's school among the jury which awarded him the prize for "Best Belgian Dance Solo". Although Cherkaoui had no formal training in contemporary dance, his talent was immediately recognized then. So he joined PARTS thereafter and became a dancer with Platel's Ballets C de la B in 1997 (see "Interview: Sidi Larbi Cherkaoui", 2008 and Dűrr, 2010, p. 19). Since 1999, Cherkaoui has worked as a choreographer with *Anonymous Society* which resulted in more than twenty productions up until now. Works such as *Foi* (2003), *Myth* (2007), and *Apocrifu* (2007) address issues of identity, cross-religious spirituality and diversity raising political debates on questions of empathy and transnational politics. Other choreographic influences on his work are Pina Bausch for her emotional quality and lyrical intensity as well as the truthful depiction of male/female interaction less harsh than the social class confrontation in Platel's work (see Cherkaoui, 2008). He also took classes in Trisha Brown's release-based movement technique which he considers valuable for its focus on "the skeleton and all the anatomy" and likewise William Forsythe's "mathematical way of structuring, [...] drawing circles with the elbow and head" (see Cherkaoui, 2008). Since 2006, Cherkaoui has been a resident artist with Toneelhuis in Antwerp, but he also works with ensembles and institutions such as Sadler's Wells across Europe and internationally.

In 2010 Sidi Larbi Cherkaoui founded *Eastman*, his own dance company. As a matter of fact, *Eastman* is merely the English translation of his last name which means "Arab" and is a religious title of honour received by the Cherkaoui clan in Morocco. There are two myths according to which the name either derived from the prophet or Omar, the second caliph (Dűrr, 2010, p. 19). And yet, Cherkaoui is not, strictly speaking, religious but rather interested in dance and movement as cross-religious expressions of a more universal spirituality. His work as choreographer is thus conceived of as similar to that in translation or diplomacy. In Don Kent and Christian Dumais-Lvowski's film *Sidi Larbi Cherkaoui: Dreams of Babel* (2009) Cherkaoui elaborates on this method of working with different dance styles in a mode of exchange with his partner. The exchange as a matter of give and take thus entails an ethics of change that involves as much of his own quest and development than that of his dancing partner. Cherkaoui is thus opening himself up to the influence of cross-cultural collaboration by travelling and taking in the different sociocultural environment as the film-makers accompany him on his journeys to India and China. The shared interest is one in ancestral cultures, song and dance as the conveyors of spiritual wisdom and truth. However, Cherkaoui's perspective on these forms is continuously informed by his own contemporary dance lens. Thus he does not consider himself a Kung Fu or Flamenco dancer, for example, although he learns from specialist dancers in those traditions.

Border crossings: *Zero Degrees* (2005)

Zero Degrees (2005) was Akram Khan and Sidi Larbi Chekaoui's groundbreaking collaborative dance performance, in which they investigated the idea of border crossing in its many possible meanings from actual border crossing and passport issues between Britain, India and Bangladesh, to border crossing between different cultural identities as well as life and death. Originally, the choreography evolved from establishing a bond of friendship and trust between the two performers, which Khan initially described as a way of courting and flirting with each other. This way Khan took on the more metrical counting of rhythmical sequences and layering derived from Kathak, whereas Cherkaoui was concerned for the overall integrity of meaning for the piece. In that sense, there had to be a consequential follow-up on individual moves and gestures in correspondence to the spoken section dealing with Khan's travel on the India–Bangladesh border and the encounter of a dead man on the train.

The topic of "zero degrees" thus resonates with the no space of cross-cultural existence, but also the neutral space Khan suggests his dance collaborators to start from. So whether as the son of Bangladeshi immigrants in London or the Arabic immigrant community in Antwerp, the constellation was supposed to tease out the mutual commonalities and differences between both artists in their creative process and work. Another theme derived from the idea of duality or cloning to question the nature of humanity in the twenty-first century (see Sanders, 2007). Both dancers were, for example, interested in the moment where one becomes two which is also taken up by Antony Gormley's two silicone mannequins present on stage for the entire time (in Khan 2008, DVD booklet, p. 7). Another philosophical strand of the choreography is, lastly, the journey from life to death and the responsibility one takes as an individual facing existence on those existentialist terms. The dance therefore becomes a crucial lesson in identity and cross-cultural understanding.

The performance opens with the empty stage and two white dummies cast by Antony Gormley downstage left and upstage right lying flat on their backs with face to the ceiling, feet flat footed up against the side walls and arms extended to the sides halfway between shoulders and pelvis. As an audience, we may not know that these casts were created from the living bodies of the two male dancers, Akram Khan and Sidi Larbi Cherkaoui, they could be mere visual arts sculptures, aesthetic objects as such. If, however, one knows about Antony Gormley's visual art, one may discern that perhaps the two casts are concerned with his artistic concern for redefining the meaning of sculpture in the public space, not so much as a celebration of heroism but contemplation upon the vulnerability of the human body. Gormley's concern for verticality in the face of gravity would thus be one that he shares with dance and perhaps the reason he approached Akram Khan for collaboration on one of his dance pieces in the first place. Thus, Khan reports, in the interview accompanying the performance DVD, that Gormley's initial interest to work with both dancers on this project derived from their common love of the human body.

The phenomenology of love and friendship draws a line from Aristotle through to Martin Heidegger (1889–1976), Hannah Arendt (1906–1975) and Hans-Georg Gadamer (1900–2002), and personal love usually references a person one loves for their own sake. If one were to postulate a love for dance, then this love would simply mean that one loves to dance for the sake of dance. Such transfer from a love of another person to the love of dance means first of all an engagement with loving oneself in the act of dancing. Dancing together hence enables the two dancers, Akram Khan and Sidi Larbi Cherkaoui, to share their love for dance as a common ground upon which the two of them meet, when they enter the stage from the wings left and right. In synchrony both dancers step decidedly forward and stop centre stage where they sit down in a cross-legged thinking pose close to the audience. Both of their hands are loosely folded onto each other as the left palm covers up the right hand and both elbows are placed upon the knees such that the chin and entire head may rest on top while slightly bent to the right side with eyes cast down to perhaps suggest brooding over something. The use of the hands is crucial and introduces one of the leitmotifs of the dance, as the hands, very much like traditional Indian mudras, are used to lure in the audience to empathetically partake in the emotional energy expressed by the work which blends aesthetic strategies from Kathak with European contemporary dance forms.

In his article on "Rasaesthetics" Richard Schechner has talked about the difference in approach between Aristotelian and Indian aesthetics by analysing the main dramaturgical principles of the *Poetics* and the *Natyasastra*. It thus appears that Akram Khan and Sidi Larbi Cherkaoui's collaborative choreography works with both aesthetics in a combination of visual-analytic and emotive-affective strategies. As Schechner explains,

> The presence and location of ENS [Enteric Nervous System] confirms a basic principal of Asian medicine, meditation, and martial arts: that the region in the gut between the navel and pubic bone is the center/source of readiness, balance, and reception, the place where action and meditation originate and are centered. A related place is the base of the spine, the resting spot of kundalini, an energy system that can be aroused and transmitted up the spinal column. Gaining an awareness of and control over the gut and lower spine is crucial to anyone learning various Asian performances, martial arts, or meditations. (2001, p. 38)

Khan himself has commented similarly that his interest is as much with the emotive expression of dance as with its analytic–scientific aspects (see Barnes, 2005). Schechner further emphasizes how traditional Asian performance makes use of the hands to guide the audience inside the expressed emotion, which may or may not be felt by the performer, but becomes communally shared in the theatre space (2001, p. 46). He explains,

> The rasic performer opens a liminal space to allow further play – improvisation, variation, and self-enjoyment. The performer becomes a partaker herself. When she is moved by her own performance, she is affected not as a character, but as a partaker. Like the other partakers, she can appreciate the dramatic situation, the crisis, the feelings of the character she is performing. She will both express the emotions of that character and be moved to her own feelings about those emotions. Where does she experience these feelings? In the ENS, in the gut – inside the body that is dancing, that is hearing music, that is enacting a dramatic situation. The other partakers – the audience – are doubly affected: by the performance and by the performer's reaction to her own performance. An empathetic feedback takes place. (2001, p. 46)

Khan and Cherkaoui make such rasic use of their hands throughout their performance, which indeed allows the spectator a very direct emotional entry point into the narrative dimension of the story. At the same time hands and arms are prominent elements of Cherkaoui's contemporary aesthetic as well (2006, p. 49). These gestures and emphasis on hands can be thought of as contemporary mudras to convey thought and reflection (thumb and index finger holding the chin), a heartbeat (beating of chest), tenderness (an open palm caressing or holding the cheek), violence (a beating fist or slap), etc.

Accordingly, the next sequence then introduces the narrative, since Kathak is a storytelling dance, and yet the decision to verbalize thought as text appears a more contemporary theatre move than solely conveying the emotive movement pattern. Akram Khan's journey from India across the border into Bangladesh forms the underlying narrative structure, which appears in three fragments interspersed by solo and duet dances by the two performers (see Sanders, 2007). Both dancers speak in sync articulating their text not so much via the actual words being spoken but through the choreographed gestures underlining the rhythm and movement of the speech pattern. Cherkaoui's interest in working with text is thus based in the musicality and non-verbal subtext of language, which the choreography and intonation help to ennunciate. Somewhat critical of conventional acting styles, Cherkaoui finds that dance may allow for an honesty to come through seldom revealed in Western modes of stage realism (in Khan, 2008). While this focus on hands and gestures approximates the Indian dance aesthetic of mudras to create rasa for the audience, it also translates the story, which both the dancers initially used to familiarize themselves with each other, to also communicate with their contemporary audience.

In order to understand Khan's perspective, Cherkaoui started by filming his way of storytelling which ended up finding its way into the choreography in the abstracted gesture-dance just described. As said, these gestures are mostly focused on the elaborateness of hands held together fingers intertwined, or a finger pointing at the audience in direct address underlined by a straight forward confronting look. But they also are hands pointing at the eyes with index and middle finger forming a v-shape as if to suggest a magnifier to better see through you and become more threatening, when thinking of those border guards staring at you, while they take your passport with them which may or may not be returned to you. As the actual story then talks about Khan's encounter with the border guards between India and Bangladesh, the way that their soulless look would reveal power and how a human being's identity was all of a sudden only accounted for via the piece of paper called a passport signifying either British (red passport) or Bangladeshi (green passport) citizenship. The encounter appears disturbing for the sense of exposure and vulnerability felt, where one's identity is reduced to holding a passport and the anxiety of handing it over to the guards and being at the whim of their power. It also speaks of the arbitrariness of birth and location, the difference a mere piece of paper may make between a good and a bad life as well as a sense of the possibility and threat of death overshadowing life at any moment.

At the end of this first sequence, both dancers stand up and stay on each side of the centreline drawn across the dance floor. They stop in the middle of the stage, each remaining on his side of the line, facing each other and starting a dance that evolves from the initial composition of shared gestures into a free-flowing dance of encountering arms and hands dancing with each other from across the line. The stage spotlights are soft and dimmed and focus on the two pairs of arms, their difference in shape and color, where a light brown skin meets with a pale beige skin mutually entangling each other leading into a duet that flows across their individual boundaries until the two arms become four and merge into a single entity of yet another dancing being of arms and torsos reminiscent of four-armed Indian Gods such as Vishnu or Shiva. Their God-like dance thus dissolves the separation they initially set up by sitting down as the two dancers narrating Khan's story. It is interesting to observe the invasion of the solo dancer's kinaesthetic sphere in this instance, for as Royona Mitra comments this is against traditional Kathak convention. While Mitra claims that this space of the extended arms and erect spine would never be invaded in the classical repertoire, the intertwining of the two dancers marks a crossing of boundaries whereby the dancer is no longer constructed as "pure and abstinent" but physically and emotionally involved (2009, p. 57). Hence, the duet expresses an openness to share the dance experience more directly not only with each other but also for the audience. Their shared energy and contact allow for the free flowing of energy to mark an encounter between equals beyond the discursive rules and regulations of borders and passports until the dance of intertwined arms ends and both dancers quickly withdraw towards each sidewall in the dark. The godliness of the dancers themselves appears to become the point rather than an expression of traditional Kathak aesthetic.

When they next come back to the line, the dance becomes more daring with Khan stepping over into Cherkaoui's dance territory and finally both of them cross over and change sides. While the choreographic pattern appears to mirror the combat between two virtuoso dancers engaging in some sort of danced border contest, it also opens out into the wider space as the scenography and light-change cast four simultaneous shadow doubles on the side and back walls. Kathak's stylistic prominence here consists in referencing the body's vertical line and fast spinning circles forever opening up into infinite space, where the two bodies intriguingly merge into one giant shadow figure looming large on the back wall. At the same time, the actual performers remain separated on the two sides, appearing seemingly tiny by comparison, so that only their enlarged shadows hold hands at first, and then merge into one large shadow out of which a single shadow separates continuously spinning outward.

The shadow play's beauty consists in the two-dimensional image of the black bodies cast upon a blue–grey wall as a visual effect that evokes a lifelessness similar to Antony Gormley's white casts on the floor, even though the shadows spin ever so fast while the body casts lie forever so still. The blue–grey may indeed evoke the colour of "Karuna" (pigeon colour) which according to the *Natyasastra* evokes the rasa of compassion and pathos resulting from sadness and grief (Rangacharya, 1986, p. 39). The choice of colour symbolism is important as the ghostly white of Gormley's casts invokes an ancestral belief system by which ghosts are usually painted in white. Both Khan and Cherkaoui have reflected upon the powerful experience of being entombed during the making of the casts so that their physical presence on stage indeed evokes an image of eternal time as it is represented by sculpture in its stone-like lastingness but also in the extreme expenditure of energy by the ever-so quickly spinning dervish-like Kathak dancer.

Indeed, sculpture and dance, one may say, allow for a premonition of infinity. As we all know, it is of course impossible and quite foolish to chase after one's own shadow and yet it is forever so clearly perceived by everyone under the sun, as well as on the theatre's back wall here: shadows exist, only that we cannot say where. At the end of the shadow dance Khan's extended arm strikes Cherkaoui to the floor using his hand as a tool to touch, but also kill. As Cherkaoui lies lifeless on the floor, he becomes a direct visual clone of his body cast. Khan retreats directing his look at his hands as if to question: "What have I done?" – only to then keep on spinning with hands held up above his head extending all the way up from his shoulders reaching towards the ceiling.

The music fades as Cherkaoui lifts his right arm from the elbow stretching out his hand with all fingers while still lying flat on the ground. Khan moves over as if glad to see him still alive, but as he further attempts to take his friend's hand, Cherkaoui retreats by pulling back the arm. Finally, as Cherkaoui's hand slowly reaches over to the left shoulder, Khan picks up the impulse to assist him rolling over on top of his belly. Cherkaoui lies there visibly breathing until Khan touches his spine just below the shoulder blades to trigger Cherkaoui's rapid lifting up from the ground into embryo pose. As Khan's fingers move down the single vertebrae of the spine, Cherkaoui moves up and down puppet-like transforming himself into a dribbled play ball of Khan's will. Then he moves by his volition, but still as if guided by attached strings like a marionette.

This sequence suggests an exploration of what it is that makes us move in the first place: the spine, somebody else pushing us at will or dragging us along or making us stand up, and yet ever so often we may still fall through not carrying our own weight. And so, Cherkaoui, as well, keeps falling into the floor until he lies next to his body cast again in the exact same pose with feet against the wall. Thus the play between Khan and Cherkaoui makes us question the difference between the human body and the two plaster casts until Khan moves Cherkaoui's cast away from him, and puts it centre stage for closer scrutiny and examination by performers and audience.

Dancing body and sculpture

Antony Gormley's sculpture explores the human body at the intersection between the inside and outside, the visible and invisible. His body casts inhabit different postures from lying, standing and sitting very much as a modern or contemporary dancer may explore similar positions. These postures are derived from Gormley's Buddhist inspired aesthetic, which conceives of these postures as meditative "mental states" (Craiger-Smith, 2010, p. 31). It was consequently during his three years in Asia and India, in particular, that Gormley discovered sculpture, because according to his own words it "deals with the real, and is not about making illusion or pictures isolated from the world by a frame. It is about being in the world" (in: Craiger-Smith, 2010, p. 10). Hence, the two essential qualities of his sculpture are stillness and silence, which were then also explored by Khan and Cherkaoui during their choreographic process. While the connotation of such contemplative iconicity evokes religiosity, the work as such is a-religious in its abstraction, which may evoke images of the Buddha, Hindu gods, Christ or Mohammed.

Gormley, who not only constructed the body casts but also created the spatial choreography, thereby mirrors the dance's expressivity in the visual artist's concern over a "tension between the perception of a body within space and that of a space within the body" (Schneckenburger, 2007, p. 63). As Schneckenburger further describes,

> Gormley brings out the body consciousness that develops from casting observation inward. We remember his three-year stay in Asia, especially in India, where he discovered Buddhist meditation, which he later integrated into his work. This alone should keep us from emphasizing the claustrophobic interpretation too strongly. In reality, the artist aims at an inward 'Phenomenology of the Body' (Merleau-Ponty) in a much more fundamental sense. (2007, p. 63)

In this respect Antony Gormley's collaboration influenced the entire choreographic process, as the creation of the casts became somewhat of a second birth for both performers, not too easy to deal with during rehearsal as Khan confessed. Only when the dummies were given names – in Khan's case the reversed of Akram "Marka" – was a dance with the dummy made possible. Likewise, Cherkaoui's following solo with his own dummy refers to the idea of how we often feel ourselves victim to others, when really we are only victim to our own destructive habits (see Khan, 2008).

This sequence sets in with a drumbeat underlying Cherkaoui's beating against his own chest as if to symbolize the heartbeat from within providing the tact to his movement. His solo unfolds in front of his upright positioned body cast thus establishing a danced dialogue between them as if to interrogate his alter ego indirectly commenting on notions of the self, the fact of upright posture and the erect spine as our evolutionary marker of what it means to be human. Interestingly enough, however, Cherkaoui' s dance remains firmly tied to the ground, crouching and floating in embryonic flexing and contortion of the spinal column reminiscent of yogic asanas. Repeatedly he stands on his head to reverse the flow of energy and thus questions the origin and derivation of human logic. In *Pèlerinage sur soi* (2006) Cherkaoui comments upon how he encountered the benefits of yoga during his collaborative working process with Akram Khan taking Iyengar yoga class with Sri Louise at the time (2006, pp. 31–32). Essentially, the solo appears to reference what is often referred to as the subtle body by making use of chakra energy coiled in the lower sacrum and referred to as the source of creative energy, mysticism and imagination (see Vivekananda, 1914). As opposed to the erect stance of human evolution and self-affirmation, his dance becomes a deconstruction of self and identity affirming the yogic no-self as a powerful connector between heart energy, spirituality and mind. At the same time, Khan, who remains to the side, approaches his dummy, sits on his legs and pulls up the dummy's arm to rest his head in the dummy's soothing palm. If the dummy in this instance represents the ego, then it suggests how we hold on to its functional controlling mechanism and soothing comfort. Thus, at the end of his solo, Cherkaoui gets up and stands opposite his dummy confronting its look, shaking his alter ego's hand, tapping on its shoulder, caressing the plaster cheek, hitting and finally strangling it. All of his movements thus symbolize the all-too familiar struggles of identity in crisis.

In a way this almost comic self-confrontation represents the level on which identity-discourse operates, because it is based on a Western notion of egocentric appropriation and domination of self but also others. It is on the level of self that we seek private possessions, recognition, and property rights often at the detriment of those who are in a less powerful position. Yet, at the moment of crisis, the dance may suggest an alternative route by pointing a way out of the self. In the choreography this switch takes place by Khan stepping onto his alter ego starting to recite Kathak bols for Cherkaoui to repeat. Cherkaoui, who likewise steps onto his body cast (or false notion of ego) responds and together the two dancers give over to the rhythmic pattern.

Apart from their brief training with PARTS in Brussels, the two dancers also share a love for Bruce Lee and Kung Fu films. Thus, this section layers martial arts vocabulary as a shared movement idiom on top of the Kathak derived rhythmic pattern. The emotion conveyed by the motions here appears rather more aggressive, perhaps the confrontation of two male egos, which may appear somewhat reminiscent of the atmosphere at the India-Bangladesh border patrol. The spectator may enjoy the virtuosity of the movement itself as a spectacle, just as we would enjoy an action movie, and yet there is a discomfort stressed by the abrupt pauses as to what the outcome and consequences of the fight may be. Cherkaoui and Khan do not go that far, but at the end, when Cherkaoui touches the head and heart of his dummy, puts him up and embraces him, it seems suggestive of the destructive force of ego and how our emotions – positive and negative, loving and aggressive – derive from a complex interplay of heart and mind and moving energy.

The choreography then picks up the story from the beginning, and this time Cherkaoui narrates the events from Khan's journey. So eventually, Khan's passport was returned and together with his cousins he embarked on the connecting train journey to Calcutta. While the journey itself is portrayed as a dance choreography using many turns across the diagonals to associate the free-floating enjoyment of travelling itself, the mood switches towards utter stillness and silence as Cherkaoui sits down on Kahn's bent legs. In this unified position, both dancers narrate the story about the traumatic encounter of the dead man on the train, as well as the helplessness felt towards his mourning wife. As she cries out for support, people refuse to help her carry the man off the train fearing bureaucratic hassles. At this point the atmosphere of the dance changes again into a deeper exploration of sadness and lament, embodying the grieving over a dead person. Royona Mitra's analysis of *Zero Degrees* points out that Khan chose "the use of pure Kathak abhinaya (a Sanskrit term from the *Natyashastra* that means theatricality associated with characterization), and danced to the Urdu lyrics of a young bride mourning the loss of her lover" in order to convey his vulnerability and helplessness in recalling the memory of the dead body (2009, p. 51). The sequence is tender and sorrowful as it slowly grows into a prayer, which Khan recites from the Qur'an. Cherkaoui joins in, moving towards him and beginning to weep as he drags one of the casts forward carefully putting him downstage by arranging one arm forward and putting the head to the side, whereby he instigates a ceremony of communal mourning. Essentially, the entire dance becomes a form of meditation deeply investigated in the energetic core of an emotional field surrounding the ontological question of life and death.

Khan's perspective on choreography as expression is crucial for it redefines earlier divisions in contemporary dance by bringing emotion and analysis back together again. As a matter of fact, they are always working towards the same end, if considered from a yogic spiritual perspective, which ultimately dissolves such binary. If we take yoga to simply present a spiritual quest, then it may appear useful to mark the underlying aesthetic sensibility of *Zero Degree*s, because similar to Gormley's sculptural work it allows for a cross- or even a-religious perspective reverberating across mystic traditions in Buddhism, Christianity and Islam. Swami Vivekananda's *Raja Yoga*, for example, distinguishes various yogic paths towards freedom among them the so-called Jnana (philosophy), Karma (self-less work) and Bhakti (love) paths. These paths, according to early Vedanta philosophy, reunite in freedom from self or in higher love which is also the goal towards which knowledge is directed. Such love embraces compassion for all living beings and souls, and it involves a practice of empathy. Gormley's sculptural work certainly invites such empathy, because the iconic stillness of his body casts challenges the spectator to enter into a relational engagement. There are several moments in *Zero Degrees* where this sensibility of his work is also becoming a key entry point for the audience.

The most engaging is perhaps the sequence towards the very end. After Khan's emotive mourning solo for the dead man on the train, a more analytic reflection upon the event begins, when he continues the storytelling: "The train door, shuts, we're on our way [...]" finally reaching Calcutta central station. At this point, Khan admits that he just wanted to get to the hotel, desperate for the comfort and conveniences of the Western cosmopolitan lifestyle. And yet Khan acknowledges how utterly meaningless such comfort appeared in the face of death bringing home to him his mother's words that a human life means nothing and yet everything under the circumstances of a different country, where different rules apply. Khan's inner turmoil during the narration is ingeniously picked up by Cherkaoui's staccato relevé on-pointe in the back, which seems to embody an effort of keeping balance and posture at all costs, when really the façade of holding it together, so to speak, is going to crumble any minute. In another instant of empathy therefore, Cherkaoui decidedly steps out of the relevé into a walk downstage, taking off his shoes to then lure Khan into yet another ploy of intricate foot work on the floor counting out the beat patterns.

Of course, the complications of life will not be simply danced away like this, but the sequence may suggest that dancing again can offer a different kind of solace and reconciliation with the overall meaning of life and death. Thus, the dance duet indirectly addresses the corpse from the train in its metaphoric presence as staged by Gormley's body cast downstage. In a tangential alignment towards the cast, both Cherkaoui and Khan readdress the cast, and while Cherkaoui picks up his dancing shoes from beside the cast to take them off, Khan first points at the cast and then struggles to maintain the vertical line as his body time and again gives into the pull of gravity as he exasperatingly collapses into and lifts up from the floor. Finally though, he gives into gravity remaining still, lying flat on his belly, head turned away and arm stretched out forward in an exact mirror pose of the cast: two corpses, so to speak.

In response, Cherkaoui, who has meanwhile put on his dancing shoes, lifts one more time into the previous relevé on-pointe as if to say that all of this is just that little bit too much to deal with in an attempt of keeping risky balance here. And yet, again he will decidedly step out of it walk towards Khan and seek a way out of the dilemma by firstly examining the nature of these two unlikely corpses on stage. Are they really dead? He taps with his toe onto Khan's head, which switches direction, and then moves over to the body cast, stepping flat footed – and far less carefully – onto the body cast's spine which due to the silicone material gives in and bounces immediately back, a movement that Khan imitates simultaneously thereby establishing a direct link between his body and the body cast. The disrespectful examination and maltreatment of the body cast and Khan's imitation of the reaction presents an image of the undignified treatment of the dead man on the train, while at the same time questioning the difference we would make between a living and a dead body. Just because a body is still, does not mean that it does not continue to live and should be respected therefore. As Cherkaoui drags Khan and his dummy along the stage, and puts them both up on his shoulder as if to measure their weight, he becomes a scale for humanness in the face of death. How much does a life weigh? What is a life's worth in the world today? Too much for one man to bear, the scenic image seems to say, when both Khan and the body cast drop down to the floor from Cherkaoui's shoulders. And yet, they cannot just lie there so Cherkaoui connects Khan to both dummies and then tries to drag all of them along the floor, but yet again the weight is just too heavy.

Only towards the very end then does Cherkaoui pick up his own dummy as if to finally embrace his alter ego once again, before he sits down, places the dummy's head in his lap and starts to sing a mournful song. Interestingly, the language for the song is Hebrew, because both dancers found the reverberation to cross yet another linguistic line intriguing (2006, p. 53). This final sequence appeals to a yogic reading again, because even if we wanted to carry the whole load, all we can ever do is embrace our own little self compassionately. That way we will not only be able to cross our own boundaries of self-perception, but also allow ourselves to reach out towards other people more openly. Only in addressing ourselves can we thus reconcile our follies and failures so that we may ultimately be redeemed. Such a gesture of redemption, it appears, is also performed by Khan during this final scene, where he acts from behind his dummy standing with both hands covering the body cast's mouth. His Kathak arms and hands articulate the silence from inside Gormley's body casts, because perhaps one cannot really speak of the pain that was felt, but rather express the intensity of such emotion in dance. Khan's Kathak inflected hand mudras thus allow for such pathos to be shared empathically with the audience. Empathy is therefore a shared kinaesthetic feeling rather than intellectual understanding, even though intellect and emotion are not mutually exclusive. Similarly, it is not necessary to understand the lyrics of Cherkaoui's song, since the intonation communicates straight to the listener's heart where it reverberates internally but also externally.

The emotion of sorrow fills the entire theatrical space at this point and ignites Khan's shaking tremble all the way through his body into our own marrow and bone. It is again in line with rasaethetics and the yogic teachings here that one partakes in emotional energy via an inside/outside feedback loop. The godly within our own body speaks of a higher love and compassion that connects each cell of the human body with the entire universe. And yet to make the realization, it is not necessary to change the world, but only to address one's own foibles, the vulnerable, resisting dummy we each carry within ourselves. Following a yogic reading of the performance, *Zero Degrees* ultimately becomes a dance-meditation on friendship and love for their endless capacity to teach us human compassion and empathy. Such empathy is at the heart of Gormley's sculpture, but is also in the collaborative sharing process between Khan, Cherkaoui and the musicians behind the gauze. Throughout the piece, the emotional quality is transported by the music and singing. It creates the rasic impact of Karuna and its sorrowful atmosphere for contemplation. Eventually though, the dance overcomes this sadness as it enables the dancers to share their

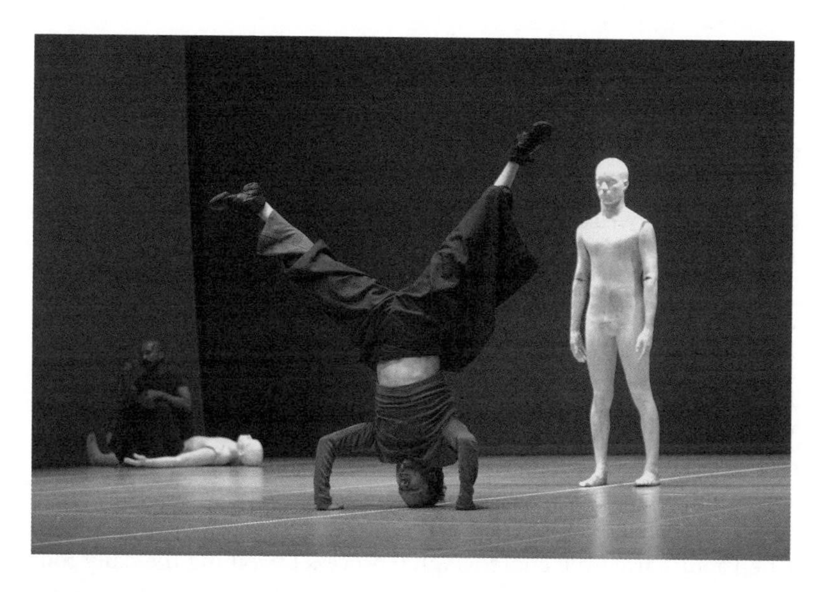

Akram Khan and Sidi Larbi Cherkaoui in *Zero Degrees* at Sadler's Wells © Alastair Muir.

loneliness at zero point. Dancing together, Khan, Cherkaoui and their ghostly dummies, merge into one larger than life figuration of humanness so that at the very end the two lonely casts take on yet another life, as they remain silent on stage, while both actors exit the scene.

Sidi Larbi Cherkaoui: *Sutra* (2008)

Cherkaoui's award-winning choreography *Sutra* (2008) picks up on many of the themes already explored in the earlier collaboration with Akram Khan and Antony Gormley and becomes exemplary of Cherkaoui's ongoing quest and exploration of spirituality in his work. The early influence of yoga, vegetarianism and meditation pointed the path, which took Cherkaoui towards China and the Shaolin Temple in May 2007. Thus, Cherkaoui, the ardent admirer of Bruce Lee's Kung Fu films, first met Master Shi Yongxi intending to observe his Kung Fu and T'ai Chi martial arts doctrine as taught and practised by the Shaolin warrior monks living there today (see Szporer, 2009). While Cherkaoui was taking a breather from the extensive touring circuit, the monks, likewise, shared an interest in an artistic encounter that could present an alternative to the virtuosic Shaolin touring sets and meanwhile somewhat stereotypical performance style they were presenting abroad. After extensive touring with *Zero Degrees* as well as with founding his own company after separating from Alain Platel and Les Ballets C de la B, Cherkaoui's encounter with the Shaolin ethics of conduct appeared as a welcome opportunity to recharge his creative batteries (see Mackrell 2008). In his conversations with Master Shi Yongxi then, the idea for a mutual choreography emerged, since there was an interest from the monastery to learn more about the art of dance theatre as well. As Cherkaoui comments, Master Shi Yongxi with his interest in calligraphy and the martial arts may well be considered an artist in his own right and therefore an ideal mentor for the project.

Rehearsals for *Sutra* started in January 2008 with Antony Gormley and composer Szymon Brzóska already on board as the music and scenography collaborators. During the months of February and March, Cherkaoui started the choreographic process by joining the daily routine at the monastery for meals, as well as observing and directing some of the warrior monks' training routine. However, coping with the cold proved slightly more difficult than anticipated so that Cherkaoui decided to stay at a hotel twenty minutes away and prepare with his yoga while the monks would be warming up jogging in the cold. Also, Cherkaoui preferred rehearsing in hat and gloves to protect his body from injury, while he was learning some of the Kung Fu movements himself. Despite some similarities to his dance vocabulary therefore, Cherkaoui also quickly observed the dangers that an untrained body may encounter upon merely imitating the formal aspects of the Kung Fu style. He comments,

> Everything they do is very beautiful, although some of it could actually break your arm. One spiralling move was lovely in thin air, but when I did it with one of the monks, it pulled me almost onto the floor. I'm surprised by how familiar certain moves are, as if dance elements cross cultures. There's a flipping of the shoulders the monks do, like a dolphin, that I use in my own choreography. Some jumps look more like jazz to me than kung fu. (in: Mackrell, 2008)

The majority of the monks Cherkaoui was working with were at the comparatively young age between twenty-one and twenty-two, which allowed for an easier rapport between them and the Western choreographer with only an age difference of ten years. And yet, one of the difficulties consisted in asking them to start thinking about their movement routine from a dance theatre perspective. Likewise, Gormley's three-wall empty box structures were part of the rehearsals from the very beginning as well as Brzoska's melancholic musical score for piano, percussion and strings, which provided further challenges to structuring the overall movement alignment for the piece. Yet, because Cherkaoui's approach is very visual and in many ways very close to drawing, he started from images created by the boxes in space as much as the movement they afforded for being manipulated in different set ups. So initially, Cherkaoui suggested that the monks simply play around with Gormley's boxes similar to a game of super-size Lego (Mackrell, 2008).

Such playfulness in the encounter with the Shaolin monks is one of the key strategies Cherkaoui employs in his cross-cultural collaborations. As a dancer, he regresses into the state of a child free to play and this became part of the relationship and red thread for the later work in his interactions with the ten-year-old Shi Yandong alias "Dong Dong", a comparatively young Shaolin novice at the temple to join the project as well. Since he was not as tall, he appeared more flexible to perform Kung Fu inside Gormley's box structure. But then Cherkaoui also discovered that collaborating with Dong Dong allowed for more flexibility and openness to enter the performance, since he was more easily willing to improvise and make up little stories, which ultimately resulted in a co-creation of the entire piece (Mackrell, 2008). This youthful sensibility found its way into the performance later on with Cherkaoui and Dong Dong, indeed, manipulating a Lego-size miniature set of boxes in anticipation of the emerging lifesize box configurations on stage.

Throughout his stay at the temple, Cherkaoui was most fascinated by how effortlessly Shaolin culture would integrate the ancient Buddhist teachings and spirituality with a contemporary reality of mobile phones and internet (see Mackrell, 2008). Thus Kung Fu embodies all the essential movement qualities of the animal kingdom (tiger, dragon, horse, cat, pigeon, leopard etc.) and works in and with the natural environment (water, fire, air and rock) in its vocabulary, stances and style (see Fernandes, 2002; Liuhai, 1996). The simultaneity of modernity and tradition thus became one of the initial ideas for the performance. Although the actual man-size boxes are made of three plywood walls, a concept Gormley had already explored in earlier sculptural work such as Allotment 11 (see Martin, 2007), the swift ease with which the quite heavy (32 kg) boxes were eventually manipulated by the monks makes one question the entire concept of their materiality, form, force and dynamic. The boxes thus translate for us the mysterious force underlying Kung Fu martial arts practice called "Chi" as it becomes evident that each living thing – material and immaterial – is interconnected and continuously shape-shifting.

Cosmic energy and body–mind

Sutra essentially refers to the original Buddhist teachings and aphorisms underlying the Shaolin martial arts. Kung Fu and T'ai Chi are thus primarily a psycho-physical discipline for obtaining enlightenment (samadhi) via a set of training postures to cultivate "Chi" which is essentially an embodiment of universal cosmic energy. As Fernandes defines,

> Chi in the broadest sense means energy. Chi is what drives the wind and gives the sun its power. It is what makes plants, animals and people grow, reproduce and flourish. Breath is chi but chi is more than just air. It is the vital force that keeps us alive. (2002, p. 196)

Intrigued by the rhythmic interchange of explosiveness and stillness characteristic of Kung Fu boxing sets, Cherkaoui explored the underlying movement system of Kung Fu in order to align it with contemporary choreographic strategies. As with all of his choreographic forms Cherkaoui was interested to break through the cliché formula of Kung Fu virtuosity in order to make the underlying spirituality that informs the work more visible to a Western audience (2008a).

Life at the monastery reverberated strongly with ideas Cherkaoui and Gormley had already explored in their previous work with Akram Khan. One of the common strands consisted in the notion of replication or cloning to emphasize a conceptualization of the human beyond notions of self-centred individualism. For example, Cherkaoui observed that out of two hundred monks at the Shaolin temple, the one hundred warrior monks would be training the exact same patterns as to replicate each other as if they were clones. Initially, Gormley's boxes served as something in-between a training tool (such as the monks will use in their daily practice, for example, ropes, swords, rocks) and a Lego super-toy with which the sixteen warrior monks improvised different set ups of mobile architecture before Cherkaoui started to choreograph.

The way Cherkaoui works shares an affinity with drawing, since he usually starts from a visual image, which is a method he derived from his early exploration of art and painting (2008a). Similar to film editing then, Cherkaoui selects different images from the rehearsal process to rearrange them later in accordance with the musical score and movement. However, the different types of movement performed with the box structure may also change the initial image-idea and create the possibility for new narrative content to emerge at any stage of the process. While in one image the boxes form a lotus, they become a vessel, ship or skyscraper later in the performance. Cherkaoui worked with Dong Dong's imaginary, who, because he was still a child, would more willingly delve into a world of fantasy and fairy tale. His intuitive movements allowed him to perform Kung Fu inside the box, but also to transform himself more convincingly into a little monkey, for example. As Cherkaoui commented, Dong Dong became a very strong influence for the choreography, especially in their duet. Ultimately, their collaboration suspended the hierarchical choreographer/dancer division as they became co-creators (see 2008a).

The performance begins with all of Gormley's boxes turned upside down with the open side towards the floor, thereby forming a stage platform with a Chinese jian sword stuck in the centre so that only half of it with the red tassel facing up sticks out. The jian counts as "The Gentleman of Weapons" in Chinese martial arts, also sometimes referred to as "t'ai chi sword", for the mythic connection to the bodhisattva Manjusri (Chinese: Wenshu) who is often depicted with a jian representing "the sword of wisdom" (see Sayama, 1986). While all the stage lights are initially off, the first lights go on up above Cherkaoui and Dong Dong, who sit opposite each other in lotus upon another box, which however unlike all the other boxes is not made from wood but metal. At first the two performers observe the mini stage model of Gormley's set design as if they were starting a game of chess. Then Cherkaoui moves one hand with a pointed index finger through the air pointing above the stage set, as the first warrior monk enters the stage and lifts up the sword to perform a first few Kung Fu moves across the wooden boxes until finally the other warrior monks, who are hiding underneath the boxes, will one by one, turn each row of boxes upside down with the open side facing the ceiling as if touched by the magic force of the sword. The sword as an emblem of wisdom thus symbolizes the internal essence of traditional Kung Fu arts, which is essentially an action meditation emphasizing the aspect of self-defence rather than outright attack.

Shaolin warrior monks are only partially ordained monks who take five lay precepts (no killing, no stealing, no sexual misconduct, no wrong speech and no intoxicants) in the beginning to add five more precepts once they stay on the grounds of the monastery, including full celibacy. Buddhism (= investigation of Chan) and Kung Fu (= warrior skills) training are thus mutually informative as they shape the Shaolin warriors' formation as part of Shaolin monastic life. The etymology of Kung Fu furthermore translates into "hard work" in English and refers to the idea that the power and strength of the warrior are only achieved via rigorous discipline over time so that it may carry the meaning of accomplishment and merit as the result of continuous effort and dedication. Lifelong Kung Fu practice therefore involves a deeper investigation and engagement with Chan Buddhism, which ultimately involves a deeper understanding of one's true self (see Hershock, 2005 and Sayama, 1986). The legendary sources of Chan Buddhism date back to the year 526/7, thirty-two years after the monastery was founded, when the South Indian Buddhist monk Bodhidharma (Chinese: Damo) first arrived in China to introduce his teachings on "vast emptiness" and meditation there (see Fernandes, 2002). Upon his first visit, so the legend goes, Bodhidharma withdrew to a cave on top of one of the mountains close to the Shaolin monastery where he meditated for nine years opposite a wall until his features were engraved upon it. This testimony is still kept in his memory at the Shaolin monastery today in form of that rock engraving. Despite the fact that the myth is highly contested by contemporary martial arts historians, it still appears to inform much of the spirituality underlying Kung Fu practice and its mythic appeal and proliferation in global pop culture.

Hence, the performance continues as a danced investigation of Chan-mind through the eyes of the Western choreographer and his child-ally Dong Dong, who becomes somewhat of a younger alter ego to the choreographer's playful sensibility of the child, since both of them are still apprentices rather than masters in Kung Fu at this point. Throughout the piece Cherkaoui and Dong Dong will interfere in the set construction and always return to the miniature model to sometimes check or at other times rather marvel at the evolving configurations on stage. For the next sequence, Cherkaoui and Dong Dong step down from their metal box as to rearrange the last row of boxes upon which the single warrior monk and his sword still stand. While Dong Dong, cheeky novice that he is, steels away the sword to run off and the warrior monk disappears into one empty box, Cherkaoui picks up a wooden training staff as he assumes the role of an apprentice monk during the following sequence. Half clad in Kung Fu training suit, Cherkaoui's trousers are of the same light and loose fitting grey material as the traditional Kung Fu outfit of the monks. Yet on top Cherkaoui wears a Western-style grey jacket and corporate suit darker grey shirt underneath. The costume choice seems to suggest that he is in-between the two dress codes as much as the two worlds colliding throughout the performance.

With training staff in hand Cherkaoui balances on the edge of the boxes just like the warrior monk before him. In this sequence, the staff helps him to explore the surface and dip into the depths of the box out of which suddenly another warrior monk emerges holding on to the staff. Again, the staff appears to hold particular symbolic significance as a training tool, but also for redirecting the energy in the room and between the two performers juggling on both ends of the staff, testing their strength and superiority. Finally, the warrior monk manages to take the staff away from Cherkaoui as he investigates its power in a solo performance.

The way that the staff is manipulated appears almost as if it is an independently moving agent in the warrior monk's hands. So fast does it circle and spin that the monk shows some difficulty balancing the momentum gathered by the movement. The staff thus teaches a lesson in balancing under more severe circumstances such as standing on top but merely on the narrow edges of Gormley's upside down open box structures. All this while Cherkoaoui stands quietly observing in the back, while the monk goes through his routine until his empty hand picks up something which looks like an invisible potion, a magic drink of some sort. If Chi is the energy that is in nature and nurtures the human body from outside and within, then perhaps this is what the potion entails. Alas, the story or myth behind this sequence is not entirely clear to the audience only that we observe how the monk appears to gather strength from drinking it and dares somewhat bolder moves before he awakens another comrade from one of the boxes to hold on to the staff just like Cherkaoui did in the initial sequence before that. The staff is thus passed from one monk to the next and with it the flow of energy also wanders from one performer to the next. Accompanied by the string instruments, the entire opening scene creates the atmosphere of an awakening or a ritualistic gathering of energy as one monk after the other is awakened from his box, performs a similar solo with the staff circling and swirling about him, while gathering an invisible magic potion to drink and strengthen the body.

The next sequence then introduces the idea of the "maze", which the monks construct at the same time that Cherkaoui works on his miniature model. As Antony Gormley commented, it is thus never quite clear who manipulates whom, or if, indeed, the boxes themselves carry an inner movement structure (or Chi) that only reveals itself via creative engagement (see 2008a). To a marching beat, the maze is quickly set up and Dong Dong is the one to perform his little rabbit run through at the end of which he performs a few flic-flacs (back handsprings) quickly across the front stage. Because of the melancholic piano tune, the entire hide-and-seek motif of Dong Dong searching his way through the maze and sticking up his cute little head becomes an aphorism on youth and playfulness and finding one's way through difficulty.

Next then, the maze is quickly deconstructed as the monks drag almost all boxes to both sides with only Dong Dong's remaining vertically oriented open side to the audience centre stage. The little rabbit, he performs, is trapped now, not able to move swiftly but bumps his head several times. There is not enough space, only as Cherkaoui orients the box vertically from the outside are different postures and positions enabled again, but still there is no way out. Dong Dong's movements get more frantic as he keeps slamming his palm against the three wooden walls and the anxiety is clearly communicated as Cherkaoui, assisted by one of the warrior monks, turns the entire box upside down again to burry Dong Dong underneath.

Then all the monks bring back together all the boxes into a single catwalk stage in the centre of the space. The monks assemble on both sides, then step onto the catwalk and form a single line starting a Kung Fu boxing set beginning with the common salutation known as "Amituofo". As a greeting ritual "Amituofo", or the joining of palms, signifies "Buddha remembrance" and suggests his presence to all by focusing one's concentration upon mindfulness at this moment. The mere performance of the gesture becomes a form of recitation to cut through negative karma and clear the mind to awaken compassion, respect, and honourable conduct. It thereby teaches introspective insight so that the mind becomes clear and fully aware in the present. Thus, one invokes the internal Buddha nature as quoted from the teachings of Bodhidharma:

> Buddha means awareness, the awareness of body and mind that prevents evil from arising in either. And to invoke means to call to mind, to call constantly to mind the rules of discipline and to follow them with all your might. This is what's meant by invoking. Invoking has to do with thought and not with language. (http://shaolinchancity.blogspot.co.uk)

At the end of the sequence therefore, all the boxes are vertically put upside again with each open facade facing across the line opposite each other so that two rows of man-size boxes on both sides emerge and form an open aisle or walk-way. Dong Dong, as well, is released, and briefly moves into rabbit character again, holding both arms close up in front of the chest and hands flipped down.

Then, he flic-flacs along the aisle between the two rows of boxes. The monks, who were hiding inside the box, step out and behind their box to then push it forward so that each box fits right into the box before and beyond forming a single straight line. This is followed by another boxing set on both sides facing the box-wall in front and finished by quick jumping into the box and one more time out of sight so that there is a constant sensation of appearance/disappearance for the audience. A single monk remains outside the wall, while Dong Dong climbs up on top of it. The single monk performs a few boxing moves, which Dong Dong keenly observes and hesitantly imitates until the monk moves upstage around the box towards Cherkaoui who is still manipulating the miniature box set on top of his metal box. No longer showing respect, the warrior monk simply destroys the model with one sweep of the hand and then carries off the metallic box to put it up in front of all other boxes as part of the wall with the open side facing the audience.

Cherkaoui steps inside the box, which is just his height, facing the wall with his back turned towards the audience. As he turns around his own axis facing the walls, the room for expression seems minimal. Accompanied by the melancholic piano tune, the entire scene appears wrapped in sad loneliness. Cherkaoui's arms reach outside and up the box, and his hands touch the walls and their edge which surrounds him. Then he crosses one leg above the opposite knee head bent down or lifts his body up with his knees bent all the way up to his chest to reduce himself to half size hiding his face in both hands. He stands with feet up and head down inside the box and performs a split, then he stands straight up again looking towards the wall to then hyper-extend the spine backwards facing the audience with his head upside down.

Dong Dong, who was all the while on top of the box in the dark, joins Cherkaoui. A duet between Cherkaoui and Dong Dong unfolds, which is perhaps one of the most touching scenes of *Sutra*, because it epitomizes their growing relationship throughout the rehearsal process and production. Although the box does not become any bigger with both of them moving inside it now, it becomes somewhat more expansive as Cherkaoui is no longer alone. Together they change the entire meaning of Gormley's box as confinement into a space for mutual explorations of expressive freedom. In a way it seems that, as they support each other negotiating the tightness of the space, the room for creative and emotional expression grows. Because they are two now, the movement develops into more of a playful exploration between them. Dong Dong's leg will not stretch as high, for example, so Cherkaoui lifts him up. As Dong Dong repeats ever so often throughout his performance of *Sutra,* he scratches his head for lack of an idea for the next movement just before he comes up with it. The duet thus seems to suggest how together the entrapment can evolve into something rather beautiful and mutually enriching. Finally, Dong Dong stands on Cherkaoui's feet, who lies backwards in the box with his legs up, and they hesitantly join hands in a difficult act of balancing. So difficult as a matter of fact that Cherkaoui needs to flip over backwards outside the box in his next move thus disappearing into the dark outside the light beam. But not too long, for Dong Dong offers his hands to drag Cherkaoui back into the box which is now their shelter from the hostile environment in the dark outside. Lastly, the duet becomes an allegory of the growing relationship between an older and a younger brother perhaps, or father and son, as well as master and disciple. However, it is not quite clear who is teaching whom, but then that turns out to be the case ever so often in life as well that a relationship is always influenced vice versa. Eventually, Cherkaoui lifts Dong Dong up so that he can go out, while he closes himself in lifting the box up over his head to flip it over and thus burry himself underneath it. Dong Dong is now ready to get onto another journey, or rather the performance moves into the next sequence.

The next series of images evolves from similar patterning as the monks keep moving inside and outside the boxes, dragging them across space, putting them up vertically or flipping them down either side. With Dong Dong standing up on a single vertical box and all other boxes being dragged around him in a circular fashion, the boxes become leaves of a gigantic lotus flower in the middle of which Dong Dong sits cross-legged assuming the pose of a little Buddha. The metallic box transforms into a ship attacked by pirates initiating a scene very much reminiscent of a war encounter by the end of which all performers lie lifeless on the ground. Sword-play in Kung Fu serves several functions, but mainly it teaches the warrior about what is known as the "gift of fearlessness" in Chan Buddhism (Sayama, 1986, p. 98). While it is a fight to the death of either opponent, it is also always a fight confronting one's own inner enemy. As Sayama explains,

> The master swordsman approaches the life and death encounter with the psychophysical attitude called "open on all sides." Undefensive with no attachments, he is completely relaxed and concentrated in the present time and space. Because he is centered, he is capable of infinite movement and therefore has no opening. He responds according to the patterns enfolded in the implicate order. When two masters meet, the result is mutual passing. In the end interactions become finer and finer until sensing, interpreting, and responding occur naturally from a communion beyond words (1986, p. 134).

Kung Fu is thus fundamentally based on an analysis of movement patterns underlying the distribution of cosmic energy in all life forms including animals and the natural environment.

The human body is thus conceived of as a "natural weapon" with head, elbows, hands and legs providing the instruments in combat (Fernandes, 2002, pp. 57–58). For example, there are sixteen different hand postures, some of which are "ram's head", "hammer", "tiger claw", "crane's beak", "monkey hook", that are derived from close observation of the animal kingdom and natural environment. Likewise the Kung Fu stances and footwork allow for the fluid motion and transition from one stance to another practised alongside the punches, jumps and kicking routines (Fernandes, 2002, p. 50). While it is near to impossible to account for all the classical Kung Fu sets in practice today, they were all designed to either develop "external power" or "internal power" (Fernandes, 2002, p. 94). In fact, these two are therefore hardly distinct but form a subtle continuum which underlines the entire practice. As Fernandes describes,

> To the layman who knows nothing about martial arts, the sets appear to be classical dance. Many people have the misconception that they are interesting to watch, but useless in actual fighting. They don't seem to understand that behind the graceful and elegant movements lies a highly deceptive force. A Chinese boxer's techniques are fluid and flowing. He moves into his opponent from all directions. Form helps the practitioner to develop power, grace, endurance, balance, co-ordination, speed, reflexes and prepares him to overcome an opponent easily. (2002, p. 94)

Cherkaoui's choreography delves deeply into the subtle interplay of the external and internal powers at work in Kung Fu, which are particularly brought to the fore by the accompanying musical score. The emotional intensity of the music transports some of the described levelling of the performer's internal energy to the audience.

However, the miraculous workings of Chi not only underline the traditional Kung Fu patterns which imitate the animal kingdom and natural environment but also inform the materiality that underlies the construction of cities and modern society. Therefore roughly after the first half of the performance, Cherkaoui decides to dress the warrior monks in corporate suits to evoke the image of a contemporary cityscape. The boxes now become skyscrapers as the monks find their ways through the city-labyrinth by either jogging, jumping, performing saltos or kick-jumps. It is in a way the same energetic virtuosity each one of us performs on a daily basis as we move in and outside our offices and the city-street labyrinth.

The next image, then, has the monks seated in lotus shape on top of the box-skyscraper in a meditative choreography introducing some of Cherkaoui's hand vocabulary mixed with Kung Fu boxing hands. While Cherkaoui himself sits with his back turned towards the audience on the ground level, the warrior monks tower above almost facing the ceiling and evoke an image of transcendence. And yet, transcendence in the Buddhist sense is not so much about the discovery of a beyond, but merely a shift of horizon. As Peter D. Hershock has summarized such interdependent, horizonless being-in-the-world:

> If all things are seen as interdependent – a basic Buddhist teaching – then there cannot be ultimate dividing lines between mind and body or between spirit and nature. But if attending to what lies above and beyond nature and our immediate situation is not understood as crossing a metaphysical boundary in to the supernatural, but rather as a matter of dissolving our habits of exclusion and relinquishing our customary horizons for what we allow to be relevant – a process of restoring our original intimacy with all things – Buddhism can be seen as profoundly spiritual tradition. It is a spirituality devoted to erasing the fearful anguish of feeling utterly alone in this world and to resuming full presence as an appreciated and contributing part of it. (2005, p. 6)

Such horizon shifting is precisely at work in Cherkaoui's choreography. During the next sequence, the boxes turn from skyscrapers into shelves, bunk beds or mausoleum. They also are reworked into an assembly line and falling domino-set with each monk standing upside inside the falling tower. Finally, the boxes become a fortress again and the warrior monks change into their training suits. The fortress becomes the image of the temple which guards the warrior monks' secretive knowledge of body–mind. While Dong Dong is allowed inside through the doors, Cherkaoui has to remain outside leaning and listening in on the wall of boxes to learn how to communicate beyond such obstacles.

The performance ends with a final set-up, where the boxes assume the shape of several archways inside of which the warrior monks perform another virtuoso set of Kung Fu. This image concludes the cycle of stillness and destruction, chaos, creativity and re-emerging order as the cycle of life. At the very end, Cherkaoui challenges the monks to perform a last sequence as the most essentially Kung Fu-based section of the entire work. Based on the eleven traditional forms, he asks the warrior monks to perform these continuously for five minutes, which is traditionally never performed this long; it therefore enables some of the monks to enter the choreography on the third movement sequence, as some others would already stop to pause. The final scene thus becomes a movement prayer or sutra commemorating the eternal teachings of interdependency and compassion (see 2008a).

Dance theatre goes global: Towards an ethics of interdependency

The dance theatre discussed in this final section of the book proposes a global politics of friendship, love and compassion informed by secular spirituality as the source of their movement exploration. Movement improvisations and contact work allow for this energy to cross the borders of Western egocentrism as manifested by constructions of identity, nation and religion. Instead, dance in these last instances asserts a nomadic autonomy of the subject that is post-anthropocentric and tied to a sense of unity with the cosmos. In Jean-Luc Nancy's words such subjectivity does away with the Western concept of the Other by replacing it with "an ontology of being-with-one-another", when he suggests,

> [...] critique absolutely needs to rest on some principle other than that of the ontology of the Other and the Same: it needs an ontology of being-with-one-another, and this ontology must support both the sphere of "nature" and sphere of "history", as well as both the "human" and the "non-human"; it must be an ontology for the world, for everyone – and if I can be so bold, it has to be an ontology for each and everyone and for the world "as a totality," and nothing short of the whole world, since this is all there is (but, in this way, there is all). (2000, pp. 53–54)

Western democracy appears as such an unfinished project that leaves much to desire from such an outlined perspective of global interdependency beyond self-interested economic trajectories.

Africanist dance forms – informed by Ashé – share with the use of rasa in classical Kathak and Chi in Kung Fu that they convey the underlying energetic field that sustains our emotional response to the world and human consciousness within it. Dance thereby underlines and celebrates a continuum of all earthly existence with the immaterial force field that human existence partakes of. Unlike the discursive violence of Western objectification that seeks to categorize and conceptualize the oneness of all things according to the measure of the ego's willed thought-objects, dance – aligned with Eastern yogic practice and mysticism – dissolves such binaries. As De Riencourt – whose writings have been influential on both Akram Khan and Sidi Larbi Cherkaoui – stresses, Eastern mysticism and Western science have thus come closer together since the discovery of quantum physics in the mid-twentieth century (see Cools, 2008). For De Riencourt art in the Western context fulfills a mystical function whereby it allows for phenomenological bracketing that through affect grants accessibility of the spiritual plane otherwise reached by a yogi via extensive meditational practice. He explains,

> Art is the depiction of inner psychological truth as seen through features in a face, tensed muscles, a melody, a rainbow or a sunset: it is essentially the conveying of such truth by means of unique emotional participation. (1980, p. 125)

Such unique emotional participation is demanded from these choreographers, if audiences are to engage with the work on a serious level. The spectator cannot simply sit back and expect the dance to do the work of interpretation for him, but rather through intense contemplation and questioning of hegemonic order, discursive patterns and textual layers he or she will have to address the state of past violence and current politics.

Wole Soyinka's dramaturgy as well as Alvin Ailey's and Bill T. Jones's choreographic processes, on the other hand, responded to the pathos of colonialism and slavery on the African continent and in the United States by contesting the legacy of the European enlightenment promise to life and liberty for all people. The struggle for civil rights embodied by Ailey's *Revelations* in the mid-twentieth century testified to the creed of a felt desire for freedom at the heart of human existence. Freedom in terms of the moving body manifests as an energy or potential for creation. It is thus our birth right as civilians to take action and become agents of our own fate. Claims to sovereignty lie at the heart of every community, state or nation to enable a politics that organizes peaceful living together. However, under capitalist logic such living together is strictly organized by the rules of market value and is increasingly dominated by the management of finance and money. Historically, the evolution of capitalism went hand in hand with the institution of slavery. From an ethical perspective, therefore, capitalism constitutes a logic whereby the good life for some is mostly lived at the expense of others.

The prevalence of a life-affirming spiritualism that underpins the choreographic work of Wole Soyinka, Alvin Ailey, Bill T. Jones, Akram Khan and Sidi Larbi Cherkaoui hence functions as an affective mediation of dance's political claim to agency and autonomy. It establishes a civilian code of conduct that facilitates cross-cultural collaborations and diplomacy across national boundaries and cultural difference by pointing towards the immanent force of life that drives humanity's struggle to arrive at full awareness of its potential. Unlike the transnational mediation by the global media, dance theatre appears to open a public space that allows a deeper and more personal engagement with suffering at the heart of global modernity. As Stevenson emphasizes, the value of such immediate encounter is opposed to our disengagement with ubiquitous screens that mark our everyday public sphere via televised images of stereotypical Otherness:

> The television screen, in this regard, can be seen as a "door which we stand behind", rather than a "bridge" directly connecting the viewer to the sufferings of others. In this, the screen is not really a "window on the world", but can literally be seen as both a barrier between the viewer and those whose lives are represented. (2005, p. 81)

By contrast, dance theatre does not allow for such distancing unless one was to leave the theatre which by convention is harder to do for most audiences. Dance in Western theatre thus serves as the predisposition for a global civil society in the making even to those who do not yet pertain to full citizen rights in their own country. Dance theatre then becomes an open plane for phenomenological enquiry and the revision of political discourse granting the right for free assembly and speech, although that speech may yet be in the process of the moving body creating from the plane of immanence in a way still figuring out what needs to be said under the given experiential circumstances rather than merely regurgitating pre-fabricated mass media opinion and stereotypes.

Study Questions:

1. What is the relationship among dance, globalization and postcolonial performance?
2. To what extent does the dancing body become a cultural archive in post-colonial dance and theatre? Consider the political impact of kinaesthetic memory in the works of Alvin Ailey, Wole Soyinka and Bill T. Jones.
3. Consider Homi K. Bhabha's key concepts of hybridity and mimicry as tools for dance analysis. Do they help you reflect on the political impact of the choreographers discussed in this chapter?
4. What is the legacy of the countercultural revolution on the development of contemporary dance and dance theatre?
5. What is the relationship between male and female choreographers in the latter half of the twentieth century? Notice that only male choreographers were discussed in this section. Research the work of female choreographers of the same generation. Here is a list to get you started: Vincent Dance Theatre, Urban Bush Women and Jasmin Vardimon Company, but there are many more.
6. Choose a female choreographer you find interesting, and write a comparative research essay based on some of the critical issues raised in this chapter as well as drawing on some of the key concepts discussed throughout the book.

9 Phenomenological Encounters

Theatre, Dance and Human Rights

Theatre, dance and the body: Towards human rights

Dance and the body in Western theatre since 1948 demonstrate a move towards what we have come to call today the "human rights" culture (see Friedman, 2011). Human rights were declared in 1948, the same year that Helene Weigel uttered her silent scream, Antonin Artaud's radio broadcast "To Have done with the Judgement of God" was censored and Martha Graham premiered "Night Journey" – her battle cry for female sexual liberation. As we have seen in the different chapters of this book, dance is closely linked to our experience and expression of consciousness and identity. Our bodies are our windows to the world as much the eyes are windows to our soul. Indeed, bodies are our theatres of emotions, to recall Damasio's claim from Chapter 1, and so we understand our life through movement. Historically, this movement partakes in the same energy that transforms and spans across generations and countries but is never spent to recall Noether's theorem. Our energy-based body memory and soul are thus somatically linked to our evolutionary development and heritage as human species on this planet.

The Greeks who built their theatres on the slopes of mountains with a wide panoramic view ensured that the dancing circle became the centre of dramatic action. Theatre was a place to see, but it was also a place to dance, feel and empathize. Catharsis in the Western tradition derived from a notion of suffering that Aristotle's *Poetics* linked to the development of dramatic plot at the centre of which we find the Western ego. Traditionally, this was a male-dominated position focusing on the tragic heroes even if embodying a female role: Oedipus, Electra, Antigone or Kreon. In Greek theatre the characters mainly spoke or perhaps even sang, and although we know comparatively little about it, there was also dance and choreography. Tragedy thus paid tribute to human pathos and the fact that we suffer our fates rather than ever fully assume control over our lives.

If we study Western drama, we see how a lot of it has to do with the celebration of human individuation as the overcoming of fate. Dramatic heroes are usually on a quest to overcome their destiny rather than to accept the role they are given. The history of Western theatre is thus built on the evolution of the Western subject (see Fischer-Lichte, 2002). Embodiment in theatre became a vessel for self-expression on the basis of interpretation of dramatic text and emotional memory. Words became a vehicle for embodied memory, rather than the initial impulse to move based on emotional response. Phenomenology in the twentieth century, however, emerged as a critical response to Western rationalism in the aftermath of the Enlightenment in the late seventeenth century. Philosophers of the Enlightenment spurred Western modernity that introduced a body–mind split which increasingly negated the demands of the soul and allowed for the rise of fascism and totalitarianism in the twentieth century. While René Descartes was still very aware of the "passions of the soul" as the source of immanence and perception, this metaphysical connection was increasingly lost as philosophy moved into the twentieth century's two world wars and beyond.

This book started by looking at Artaud and Brecht as the forefathers of a phenomenological shift that reintroduced dance structures into theatre. Affect and passionate time, as well as gestus and scenic composition, began to choreograph the movements of actors from an embodied source of emotional memory and impulse rather than the text. Studying dramatic text in their wake therefore starts from an understanding of life itself rather than the mere study of concept and representation. While we interpret language based on our understanding of words written in the past, language bears testimony to our kinaesthetic timeshare with a historical period we ourselves have not experienced and yet sediments of which continue to live in our bloodstream and spinal cord. The fact that these words still make sense to us today testifies to the fact that the past itself lives on inside our own body. Psychology theorized this fact under the banner of the collective unconscious and archetype as the psycho-somatic structures that inform each individual life. This is to say that, fundamentally, our feelings have not changed in all these years of human evolution: pain, anger, fear and joy still feel the same, and we may even carry forward into our present some of the burden to redeem those murdered and left behind in our past lives.

Martha Graham and Jerzy Grotowski appeared very aware of such an embodied continuum as they experimented with movement techniques and impulse focusing on breathing, the spine and yogic traditions that mobilized the different energy centres of the body, when Western theatre began to dance the wrong side out again. For Graham this was a response to American society between the wars and the emancipation of women and female creativity, while Grotowski spoke to a generation traumatized by the two world wars in Europe. His quest for on organic life and a theatre of sources inspired a whole generation of theatre directors, choreographers and dancers of the 1960s who sought to bring art and life together in an attempt to change the world. They "put their bodies on the line", in Mario Savio's words, to protest the power politics of consumerism, war and nuclear extinction. While Peter Brook examined the madness at the heart of Western modernity, Richard Schechner, Judith Malina and Julian Beck resurrected the dancing chorus in their psycho-physical explorations of actor training. Postmodern dance in the wake of Merce Cunningham and Anne Halprin's pioneering efforts evolved as a critique of dance that shared similar concerns raised by the theatre practitioners of the time: how to bypass intentionality and concept in order to create dances that were closer to life and its ever pulsing creative energy? Yvonne Rainer's *Trio A* effaced all previous expectations of dance as she created continuous movement as a pertinent critique of consumerism and spectatorship.

European dance theatre emerged around the same time, and Pina Bausch in Germany as well as Anne Teresa De Keersmaeker in Belgium were both influenced by the theatre and dance that surrounded them. Their studies took them to the United States at a significant time of their development as dancer/choreographers where they picked up on the political issues and sensibilities of their time. As women, their perspective of the world shared a concern with Graham's work as a woman to create and articulate a female creative response that while not excluding men or male energy from their dance would nonetheless distinctly voice a female perspective on dance and the world. Their work influenced more contemporary choreographers, such as Sasha Waltz, as our study moved into the 1990s and the twenty-first century. Dance theatre thus emerged at a time in history when Europe moved closer together in a unification process that began 1948 and into the end of communism with the fall of the Berlin Wall 1989.

The last section of the book considered decolonization and globalization as yet another factor that impacted on dance in Western theatre with choreographers and writers such as Wole Soyinka, Alvin Ailey and Bill T. Jones. African and African diasporic dance forms survived and migrated in works such as *Death and the King's Horseman, Revelations* and *Last Supper at Uncle Tom's Cabin*. The Yoruba in Nigeria refer to Ashé as the underlying energy and life force of Africanist dance. As such it permeates all the discussed works and links them back to the origins of perhaps all dance cultures on the African continent if we consider the origin of modern Homo sapiens in East Africa. These works make a claim on human and civil rights, while putting into question the hegemony of Western rationalism and its politics of war and colonial domination. Postcolonial critiques propose that the dancing body claims its own memory and history countering Western models of domination and discourse.

Towards the end of the previous chapter I gave an outlook on the ongoing cross-cultural collaborations of Akram Khan and Sidi Larbi Cherkaoui in *Zero Degrees* (2005) and *Sutra* (2008a) as a distinctly twenty-first century perspective of interdependency in performance. Both choreographers are from a second-generation migratory background connecting the links between almost all of the traditions discussed in the book, and their open approach to collaboration speaks of a phenomenology of kinaesthetic empathy and compassion. In their early twenty-first-century work we find traces of kathak, yoga and contemporary Belgium dance, as well as Bausch's dance theatre, Chinese T'ai Chi and martial arts and even Khan's direct link to Peter Brook as he performed in *The Mahabharata*. Dance in Western theatre thus evidences the living memory of the body in performance. Throughout the many examples in this book, dance continuously projects a vision of life into the future that we already inhabit. While the final chapter solely addresses male choreographers, and I feel guilty for it, I have decided to give you the task now to investigate what women choreographers of their generation, such as Jasmin Vardimon and Vincent Dance Theatre, have been doing at the same time, and I trust that you will do this work well. No book can ever cover all the answers; these were dances I saw and now it is up to you to see and analyse more than I ever can. This is your task now to explore and write the answers I could not even think of!

Theoretically, the book gave you the tools to do so. We covered a range of phenomenological thinkers ranging from Michel Henry and

Bernhard Waldenfels to Maurice Merleau-Ponty and Jean-Luc Marion. Pathos, givenness and life determine our felt response to the world and this is manifest in each breath we take, each movement we make and the dance that we choreograph. Again, there was no space to go into the depth of their philosophical arguments, but it is for you to now pick up their original writings and explore for yourself how we may interpret their thought and let it inform our understanding of dance. We also considered writings on discourse analysis by Michel Foucault and Susan Foster for dance studies, as well as dance and identity in the writings of Judith Butler, Luce Irigaray and Helène Cixous to give you a perspective on gender, semiotics and representation. These will help you discern how the body produces and creates meaning, while it also represents power dynamics that inform our body's actions and movements. The body in Western theatre thus creates meaning from a position of immanence, but it also transcends its inner imaginal world into outward expression and meaning posing distinct ethical questions (see Cull, 2013). Embodiment hence constitutes an archive of performance and identity that we can study to learn about dance, theatre and society. Pierre Bourdieu's concept of habitus, but also Victor Turner's typology of ritual, social drama and communitas, are helpful markers to direct and guide your future studies as you embark upon your own quests and research projects.

Finally, a few words on choices and phenomenology before you embark on your own. In choosing the discussed examples, I was initially drawn by the fact that each of the works spoke to me on a fundamental level – they called for my critical response, because I sensed an intuited link around which they all cohered. Invisible at first I was guided by an unknowing-knowing that the link may be dance. But what is dance? It led me back to the body, movement, space and time, as well as the much neglected soul in Western thought. For me, dance is movement stirred by the soul and as such our inner yearning to express and communicate what really makes us move and take part in this world. Dance is our innermost felt reality, dormant like yogic *kundalini* energy with some, but wait to see when it comes alive in ecstasy to bring forth your own creative potential! The impulse to move is thus an indication of our aliveness in the world and a call to make life happen for ourselves in each moment that we live. As such, dance is the invisible-made-visible par excellence, manifesting the life force in and through theatre as the frame for perception and understanding of who we are as human beings. Theatre without dance is therefore empty as it is without life, dance without theatre is invisible because we can only see life in the face of others as no one has ever seen their own soul. As humans, we therefore fulfil our full potential only when life is lived and shared on those grounds of partaking in our human dignity by respecting the other's original life force which is their unique dance. Dance we may even say is thus an embodiment of the sacredness of life.

The human rights doctrine emerged from the shackles of two world wars, and yet, without true embodiment of a felt desire and need for human freedom and dignity, they remain empty words and paragraphs – a mere legal concept. Dance and theatre since 1948 demonstrate how the body started to dance as an expression of sacred life in the aftermath of war and destruction to help make these laws a felt reality among people. As such, dance is the soul of theatre, without it performance is deadly to recall Peter Brook's essay discussed earlier in the book. Today, such deadly theatre is ubiquitous in the media spectacles that surround us as a disembodied image that is not alive and lacks in soul, and people are increasingly isolated behind computer and smartphone screens. This book hopes to make a plea to your own investigation of the lived and felt human body in dance taking inspiration from the examples discussed here to make your own discoveries as you move away from the book and into the studio and along your own path of studies in performance.

Bibliography

Abram, David (1996) *The Spell of the Sensuous: Perception and Language in a More than Human World*, New York: Vintage.

Adams, Michael Vannoy (2008) "The Archetypal School", in Polly Young-Eisendrath and Terence Dawson (eds.), *The Cambridge Companion to Jung*, Cambridge: Cambridge University Press, pp. 107–124.

Adshead-Landsdale, Janet (1996) "Empowered Expression from Bausch and De Keersmaeker", *Dance Theatre Journal* 12:3, 20–23.

Agamben, Giorgio (2007) *Profanations*, Brooklyn: Zone Books.

Al-Saji, Alia (2004) "The Memory of another Past: Bergson, Deleuze and A New Theory of Time", *Continental Philosophy Review* 37, 203–239.

Arata, Luis O (1994) "In Search of Ritual Theater: Artaud in Mexico", in Gene A. Plunka (ed.), *Antonin Artaud and the Modern Theater*, London and Toronto: Associated University Presses, pp. 80–88.

Aristotle (1996) *The Poetics*, London: Penguin.

Artaud, Antonin (1976) *Antonin Artaud. Selected Writings*, ed. Susan Sontag, Berkeley: University of Berkeley Press.

——— (2005) *The Theatre and Its Double*, London: Calder Publications.

——— (2011) *Cahiers D'Ivry. Février 1947 – mars 1948 I Cahiers 233 À 309*, Paris: Gallimard.

Austin, J. L. (1975) *How to Do Things with Words*, Oxford: Clarendon.

Baas, Jacquelynn (2005) *Smile of the Buddha. Eastern Philosophy and Western Art from Monet to Today*, Berkeley: University of California Press.

Badejo, Peter (2009) "Peter Badejo on the Talking Drums", NT Programme for *Death and the King's Horseman* by Wole Soyinka, London: National Theatre.

Balme, Christopher (1999) *Decolonizing the Stage: Theatrical Syncretism and Postcolonial Drama*, Oxford: Oxford University Press.

Banes, Sally, ed. (1993) *Democracy's Body: Judson Dance Theatre 1962–1964*, Durham: Duke University Press.

______ (2003) *Re-inventing Dance in the 1960s. Everything was Possible*, Madison: University of Wisconsin Press.

Bannerman, Henrietta (1999) "An Overview of Martha Graham's Movement System (1929–1991)", *Dance Research* 17:2, 9–46.

________ (2010) "Martha Graham's House of the Pelvic Truth: The Figuration of Sexual Identities and Female Empowerment", *Dance Research Journal* 42:1, 30–45.

Barber, Stephen (1993) *Antonin Artaud. Blows and Bombs*, London: Faber & Faber.

——— (2013) *The Anatomy of Cruelty. Antonin Artaud: Life and Works. The Definite Research Archive*, Los Angeles: Sun Vision Press.

Barnes, Thea Nerissa (2005) "Article on Third Catalogue", http://www.akramkhancompany.net/html/akram_article.php?id=5, accessed 17 July 2012.

Barthes, Roland (1967) "Seven Photo Models of Mother Courage", *The Drama Review* 12:1, 44–55.
Benjamin, Walter (1983) *Understanding Brecht*, London: Verso.
Bergson, Henri (1920) *Mind-Energy. Lectures and Essays*, London: Macmillan.
——— (2005) *Matter and Memory*, New York: Zone Books.
Bermel, Albert (2001) *Artaud's Theatre of Cruelty*, London: Methuen.
Bhabha, Homi K. (1994) *The Location of Culture*, London and New York: Routledge.
Bharucha, Rustom (1993) *Theatre and the World. Performance and the Politics of Culture*, London and New York: Routledge.
Biner, Pierre (1972) *The Living Theatre*, New York: Horizon Press.
Blackburn, Robin (1997) *The Making of New World Slavery. From the Baroque to the Modern 1492–1800*, London: Verso.
Bogle, Donald (1997) *Toms, Coons, Mulattoes, Mammies and Bucks. An Interpretive History of Blacks in Film*, New York: Continuum.
Bourdieu, Pierre (1977) *Outline of a Theory of Practice*, Cambridge: Cambridge University Press.
Bradley, Karen K. (2009) *Rudolf Laban*, London and New York: Routledge.
Brauninger, Renate (2014) "Structure as Process: Anne Teresa De Keersmaeker's Fase (1982) and Steve Reich's Music", *Dance Chronicle* 37:1, 47–62.
Brecht, Bertolt (1949) *Mutter Courage: Modellbuch zur Auffuehrung*, Berlin: Akademie der Künste.
——— (1967) "Neue Techniken der Schauspielkunst. Über den Gestus (1949–55)", *Gesammelte Werke*, Bd 16 & 21, Frankfurt am Main: Suhrkamp.
——— (1976) *Bertolt Brecht Poems 1913–1956*, ed. John Willett and Ralph Manheim, London: Methuen.
——— (1980) *Die Antigone des Sophokles. Materialien zur Antigone*, Frankfurt: Suhrkamp.
Bremser, M., ed. (2000) *Fifty Contemporary Choreographers*, London: Routledge.
Brook, Peter (1961) "Search for a Hunger", *Mademoiselle* Nov, 50, 95.
_______ et al. (1966) "Marat Sade Forum", *The Drama Review* 10:4, 214–237.
——— (1986) "Talking with Peter Brook", *The Drama Review* 30:1, 54–71.
——— (2006) "Introduction", *Marat/Sade The Persecution and Assassination of Marat as Performed by the Inmates of the Asylum of Charenton under the direction of the Marquis de Sade* by Peter Weiss, London: Boyars.
——— (2008) *The Empty Space*, London: Penguin.
Brown, Carolyn (2007) *Chance and Circumstance. Twenty Years with Cage and Cunningham*, Evanston: Northwestern University Press.
Burt, Ramsay (1998) "Dance, Gender and Psychoanalysis: Martha Graham's Night Journey", *Dance Research Journal* 30:1, 34–53.
——— (2004) "Contemporary Dance and the Performance of Multicultural (kaash) identities", http://www.akramkhancompany.net/html/akram_essay.php?id=15, accessed 19 September 2011.
——— (2004) "Profile: Anne Teresa De Keersmaeker", *Dance Theatre Journal* 19:4, 36–40.
——— (2006) *Judson Dance Theatre. Performative Traces*, London and New York: Routledge.

Butler, Judith (1990) *Gender Trouble: Feminism and the Subversion of Identity*, London and New York: Routledge.

——— (2000) *Antigone's Claim. Kinship between Life and Death*, New York: Columbia University Press.

Butterworth, Joe and Gill Clarke, eds. (1998) *Dance Makers Portfolio*, Wakefield: Centre for Dance and Theatre Studies.

Cage, John (2004) *Silence*, London: Marion Boyars.

Carlson, Marvin (1999) "Body and Sign in *Marat/Sade*", *Assaph* 15, 9–17.

Carter, Alexandra, ed. (1998) *The Routledge Dance Studies Reader*, London & New York: Routledge.

Chaikin, Joseph (1972) *The Presence of the Actor*, New York: Theatre Communications Group.

Cherkaoui, Sidi Larbi (2008) "Interview: Sidi Larbi Cherkaoui Q & A", http://londondance.com/articles/interviews/sidi-larbi-cherkaoui-qanda/, accessed 24 July 2012.

——— (2009) "Acceptance Speech: Sidi Larbi Cherkaoui at the Kairos Prize Awards Ceremony Hamburg 15 February 2009", http://www.toepfer-fvs.de/index/php?id=837&L=O, accessed 6 August 2012.

——— and Gilles Delmas (2007) *Zon-Mai. Parcours Nomades*, Arles: Actes Sud.

——— and Justin Morin (2006) *Pèlerinage sur soi*, Arles: Actes Sud.

Climenhaga, Royd, ed. (2013) *The Pina Bausch Source Book. The Making of Tanztheater*, New York and London: Routledge.

Cohen, Bonnie Bainbridge (1993) *Sensing, Feeling, and Action. The Experiential Anatomy of Body-Mind Centering*, Northampton, MA: Contact Editions.

Cools, Guy (2008) *The Bi-Temporal Body: Guy Cools with Akram Khan (Body Language 2)*, London: Sadler's Wells Publications.

Copeland, Roger (2004) *Merce Cunningham: The Modernizing of Modern Dance*, New York and London: Routledge.

Craiger-Smith, Martin (2010) *Antony Gormley*, London: Tate Publishing.

Crow, Brian and Chris Banfield (1996) *An Introduction to Post-Colonial Theatre*, Cambridge: Cambridge University Press.

Csikszentmihalyi, Mihaly (2002) *Flow. The Classic Work on How to Achieve Happiness*, London: Rider.

Csordas, Thomas J., ed. (1994) *Embodiment and Experience. The Existential Ground of Culture and Self*, Cambridge: Cambridge University Press.

Cull, Laura (2013) *Theatres of Immanence. Deleuze and the Ethics of Performance*, Basingstoke: Palgrave.

Damasio, Antonio (2000) *The Feeling of What Happens. Body, Emotion and the Making of Consciousness*, London: Vintage.

Dasgupta, Gautam (1997) "Remembering Artaud", *Performing Arts Journal* 19:2, 1–5.

DeFrantz, Thomas F. (2004) *Dancing Revelations. Alvin Ailey's Embodiment of African American Culture*, Oxford: Oxford University Press.

De Keersmaeker, Anne et al. (2002) *Rosas/ Anne Teresa De Keersmaeker If and Only Wonder*, Tournai: La Renaissance Du Livre.

——— and Bojana Cvejić (2012) *A Choreographer's Score. Fase, Rosas Danst Rosas, Elena's Aria, Bartók*, Brussels: Mercatorfonds.

Deleuze, Gilles (2004) *The Logic of Sense,* London and New York: Continuum.

——— and Felix Guattari (1996) *A Thousand Plateaus. Capitalism and Schizophrenia,* London: Athlone Press.

DeMille, Agnes (1991) *Martha. The Life and Work of Martha Graham,* London: Hutchinson.

Derrida, Jaques (1997) *Writing and Difference,* London: Routledge.

De Vuyst, Hildegard (1996) "P.A.R.T.S.", *Carnet* April, pp. 32, 34.

Dixon-Gottschild, Brenda (1998) *Digging the Africanist Presence in American Performance: Dance and Other Contexts,* Westport, CT: Greenwood.

——— (2003) *The Black Dancing Body. A Geography from Coon to Cool,* New York: Palgrave.

Dodds, E. R. (1951) *The Greeks and the Irrational,* Berkeley: University of California Press.

Dolphijn, Rick (2011) "Man Is Ill Because He Is Badly Constructed: Artaud, Klossowski and Deleuze in Search for the Earth Inside", *Deleuze Studies* 5:1, 18–34.

Dreyfus, Hubert L. and Mark A. Wrathall, eds. (2009) *A Companion to Phenomenology and Existentialism,* Oxford: Blackwell.

Dűrr, Anke (2010) "iDance", *Kulturspiegel* 6, 16–19.

Elswit, Kate (2013) "Ten Evenings with Pina: Bausch's 'Late' Style and the Politics of Coproduction", *Theatre Journal* 65:2, 215–233.

Fanon, Frantz (1986) *Black Skin, White Masks,* London: Pluto Press.

——— (1990) *The Wretched of the Earth,* London: Penguin.

Fellmann, Ferdinand (2006) *Phänomenologie zur Einführung,* Hamburg: Junius.

Fernandes, Christopher (2002) *The Art of Kung Fu Wu Shu,* New Delhi: Karan Press.

Fischer-Lichte, Erika (2002) *History of European Drama and Theatre,* London and New York: Routledge.

Foster, Susan (1986) *Reading Dancing,* Berkeley: University of California Press.

——— (1995) *Choreographing History,* Indianapolis: Indiana University Press.

——— (1997) "Dancing Bodies", *Meaning in Motion. New Cultural Studies of Dance,* ed. Jane C. Desmond, Durham: Duke University Press, pp. 235–257.

——— (2010) "Merce Cunningham 1919–2009", *The Drama Review* 54:1, 7–9.

——— (2011) *Choreographing Empathy: Kinesthesia in Performance,* New York: Routledge.

Foucault, Michel (1970) *The Order of Things,* London: Tavistock.

——— (1972) *The Archaeology of Knowledge,* transl. Allan Sheridan, New York: Harper and Row.

——— (1977) *Discipline and Punish,* transl. Alan Sheridan, New York: Pantheon.

——— (1979) *The History of Sexuality. Vol. 1. An Introduction,* London: Alan Lane.

——— (2007) *Madness and Civilization. A History of Insanity in the Age of Reason,* London and New York: Routledge.

Fraleigh, Sondra Horton (1987) *Dance and the Lived Body. A Descriptive Aesthetics,* Pittsburgh: University of Pittsburgh Press.

Frank, Adam (2011) *About Time,* Oxford: Oneworld Publications.

Franko, Mark (2012) *Martha Graham in Love and War,* New York: Oxford University Press.

Franzke, Andreas and Gabriela Trujillo (2006) *Artaud – Ein Inszeniertes Leben*, Düsseldorf: Museum Kunstpalast.
Freud, Sigmund (1994) *Civilization and Its Discontents*, New York: Dover.
Friedman, Lawrence (2011) *The Human Rights Culture: A Study in History and Context*, New Orleans: Quid Pro.
Garner, Stanton B. (1994) *Bodied Spaces. Phenomenology and Performance in Contemporary Drama*, Ithaca & London: Cornell University Press.
Genter, Sandra (2000) "Anne Teresa de Keersmaeker", *Fifty Contemporary Choreographers*, ed. M. Bremser, London: Routledge.
Gilbert, Helen and Joanne Tompkins (1996) *Post-Colonial Drama: Theory, Practice, Politics*, London: Routledge.
Gilroy, Paul (1993) *The Black Atlantic: Modernity and Double Consciousness*, Cambridge, MA: Harvard University Press.
Gitlin, Todd (1993) *The Sixties. Years of Hope, Days of Rage*, New York: Bantam Books.
Graham, Martha (1991) *Blood Memory. An Autobiography*, London: Macmillan.
Grossman, Evelyn, ed. (2008) *50 Drawings to Murder Magic/Antonin Artaud*, London: Seagull Books.
Grotowski, Jerzy (1991) *Towards a Poor Theatre*, London: Methuen.
Guérivière, Jean (2004) *Die Entdeckung Afrikas: Die Erforschung und Eroberung des schwarzen Kontinents*, Munich: Knesebeck.
Guisgand, Philippe (2007) *Les fils d'un entrelacs sans fin. La danse dans l'œuvre d'Anne Teresa De Keersmaeker*, Villeneuve d'Ascq: Presses Universitaires du Septentrion.
Halprin, Anne (1995) *Moving Towards Life. Five Decades of Transformational Dance*, ed. Rachel Kaplan, Hanover: Wesleyan University Press.
——— (2002) *Returning to Health with Dance, Movement, and Imagery*, Mendocino: LifeRhythm.
Halprin, Lawrence (1969) *The RSVP Cycles. Creative Processes in the Human Environment*, New York: George Braziller.
Hargreaves, Martin (2004) "Rosas/Anne Teresa De Keersmaeker If and Only Wonder", *Dance Theatre Journal* 19:4, 41.
Harris, Melissa, ed. (1997) *Merce Cunningham: Fifty Years. Chronicle and Commentary by David Vaughan*, New York: Aperture.
Hecht, Werner, ed. (1982) *Materialien zu Brechts "Mutter Courage und ihre Kinder"*, Frankfurt am Main: Suhrkamp.
Hegel, Georg Friedrich Wilhelm (2004) *The Phenomenology of Mind*, Mineola: Dover.
Henry, Michel (2002), *Inkarnation. Eine Philosophie des Fleisches*, Freiburg: Karl Alber Verlag.
Hershock, Peter D. (2005) *Chan Buddhism*, Hawaii: University of Hawaii Press.
Hoghe, Raimund (1986) *Pina Bausch: Tanztheatergeschichten*, Frankfurt am Main: Suhrkamp.
Horosko, Marian (2002) *Martha Graham. The Evolution of Her Dance Theory and Training*, Gainesville: University of Florida Press.
Hunt, Lynn (2007) *Inventing Human Rights. A History*, New York: Norton.

Hutera, Donald (1999) "Bill T. Jones", *Fifty Contemporary Choreographers*, ed. Martha Bremser, London and New York: Routledge.

Innes, Christopher (1972) *Erwin Piscator's Political Theatre. The Development of Modern German Drama*, Cambridge: Cambridge University Press.

Irigaray, Luce (1985) *The Sex Which is Not One*, Ithaca: Cornell University Press.

Jackson, Naomi and Toni Shapiro-Pim, eds. (2008) *Dance, Human Rights, and Social Justice*, Toronto: Scarecrow Press.

Jannarone, Kimberly (2010) *Artaud and His Doubles*, Ann Arbor: University of Michigan Press.

Jones, David Richard (1986) *Great Directors at Work. Stanislavsky, Brecht, Kazan, Brook*, Berkeley: University of California Press.

Jowitt, Deborah (1988) *Time and the Dancing Image*, Berkeley and Los Angeles: University of California Press.

——— (1991) "Martha Graham", *The Drama Review* 35:4, 14–16.

Jung, Carl Gustav (1991) *The Archetypes and the Collective Unconscious*, 2nd ed., London: Routledge.

——— (1995) *Memories, Dreams, Reflections*, ed. Aniela Jaffé, transl. Richard and Clara Winston, London: Fontana Press.

——— (2003) *Four Archetypes*, London & New York: Routledge.

Karina, Lilian and Marion Kant (2003) *Hitler's Dancers. German Modern Dance and the Third Reich*, New York and Oxford: Berghan Books.

Katrak, Ketu H. (2011) *Contemporary Indian Dance. New Creative Choreography in India and the Diaspora*, Basingstoke: Palgrave.

Keleman, Stanley (1985) *Emotional Anatomy. The Structure of Experience*, Berkeley: Center Press.

Khan, Akram (2011) "Collaboration – Keynote Address for ISPA Congress at the Timescenter, New York", http://www.akramkhancompany.net/html/akram_essay.php?id=14, accessed 19 September 2011.

Kott, Jan (1970) *The Eating of the Gods. An Interpretation of Greek Tragedy*, London: Methuen.

Knapp, Bettina (1994) "Antonin Artaud: Mythical Impact in Balinese Theater", in Gene A. Plunka (ed.), *Antonin Artaud and the Modern Theater*, London & Toronto: Associated University Presses, pp. 89–101.

Kristeva, Julia (1982) *Powers of Horror. An Essay in Abjection*, New York: Columbia University Press.

——— (2002) *Revolt, She Said*, New York: Semiotext(e).

Kumar, Ravindra and Jyvette Kumar Larsen (2004) *The Kundalini Book of Living and Dying. Gateways to Higher Consciousness*, Boston: Weiser Books.

Kupke, Peter (1977) "Das Antikriegs-Stück", *Mutter Courage und ihre Kinder von Bertolt Brecht. Eine Dokumentation der Aufführung des Berliner Ensembles 1978*, Berlin: Brecht-Zentrum der DDR [1981].

________ (1981) *Mutter Courage und ihre Kinder von Bertolt Brecht. Eine Dokumentation der Aufführung des Berliner Ensembles 1978*, Berlin: Brecht-Zentrum der DDR.

Lacan, Jacques (1992) *The Ethics of Psychoanalysis 1959–1960. The Seminar of Jacques Lacan. Book VII*, ed. Jacques-Alain Miller, New York and London: Routledge.

——— (2006) *Écrits. The First Complete Edition in English*, transl. Bruce Fink, New York & London: Norton.

Laermans, Rudi (2010) "Impure Gestures Towards 'Choreography in General': Re/Presenting Flemish Contemporary Dance, 1982–2010", *Contemporary Theatre Review* 20:4, 405–415.

Lambert-Beatty, Carrie (2008) *Being Watched. Yvonne Rainer and the 1960s*, Cambridge, MA: MIT Press.

Lawlor, Leonard (2003) *The Challenge of Bergsonism*, London: Continuum.

Leach, Robert (2004) *Makers of Modern Theatre*, London: Routledge.

Ley-Piscator, Maria (1967) *The Piscator Experiment. The Political Theatre*, New York: James H. Heinemann.

Liuhai, Cai, ed. (1996) *Shaolin Kung-fu*, Beijing: Henan Art Publishing House.

Living Theatre (1971) *The Living Book of the Living Theatre with an Introduction by Richard Schechner*, New York: Graphic Society Ltd.

Mackrell, Judith (2008) "I Want to Stay Here Forever", *The Guardian*, 23 April, http://www.guardian.co.uk/stage/2008/apr/23/dance1/print, accessed 24 July 2012.

——— (2013) "Move Tube: Pina Bausch's Bluebeard", *The Guardian*, 15 February, http://www.theguardian.com/stage/2013/feb/15/pina-bausch-bluebeard-move-tube, accessed 25 May 2014.

Malina, Judith (1990) "Preface", *Antigone in a Version by Bertolt Brecht*, New York: Applause Books, pp. v–vii.

Manning, Susan (1993) *Ecstasy and the Demon*, Berkeley and Los Angeles: University of California Press.

Marcuse, Herbert (1998) *Eros and Civilisation. A Philosophical Inquiry into Freud*, London and New York: Routledge.

Marion, Jean-Luc (2002) *Being Given. Toward a Phenomenology of Givenness*, Stanford: Stanford University Press.

Markard, Anne (1993) "Jooss the Teacher. His Pedagogical Aims and the Development of the Choreographic Principles of Harmony", *Choreography and Dance* 3:2, 45–51.

Marowitz, Charles (1966) "Notes on the Theatre of Cruelty", *The Drama Review* 11:2, 152–172.

Martin, Francesca (2007) "Antony Gormley to Team Up Tiger-style with Shaolin Monks for Dance Piece", *The Guardian*, 7 November, n.p.

McDonagh, Don (1973) *Martha Graham. A Biography*, London: David and Charles.

Meisner, Nadine (1997) "Circular Moves: Continuity and Change in the Work of Anne Teresa De Keersmaeker", *Dance Theatre Journal* 13:4, 10–13.

Merleau-Ponty, Maurice (1968) *The Visible and the Invisible*, ed. Claude Lefort, Evanston: Northwestern University Press.

——— (2004) *Phenomenology of Perception*, transl. Colin Smith, London and New York: Routledge.

Mink, Janis (2000) *Marcel Duchamp 1887–1968. Art as Anti-Art*, London: Taschen.

Mitra, Royona (2009) "Dancing Embodiment, Theorizing Space: Exploring the 'Third Space' in Akram Khan's Zero Degrees", *Planes of Composition. Dance, Theory and the Global*, ed. André Lepecki and Jenn Joy, London: Seagull Books, pp. 41–58.

——— (2015) *Akram Khan: Dancing New Interculturalism*, Basingstoke: Palgrave.

Molik, Zygmunt and Giuliano Campo (2010) *Zygmunt Molik's Voice and Body Work. The Legacy of Jerzy Grotowski*, London and New York: Routledge.

Moore, Thomas, ed. (1989) *The Essential James Hillman. A Blue Fire,* London & New York: Routledge.

Morris, Gay (2001) "Bourdieu, the Body, and Graham's Post-War Dance", *Dance Research* 19:2, 52–79.

Morrison Brown, Jean, Naomi Mindlin, and Charles H. Woodford, eds. (1998) *The Vision of Modern Dance*, 2nd ed., London: Dance Books.

Müller, Bettina (2011) "Körper, S, and noBody, a trilogy by Sasha Waltz", DVD booklet, Berlin: Arthaus Musik.

Murray, Jan (2005) "Agent Provocateur", *Dance Australia* 138 June/July, 20–21.

Nancy, Jean-Luc (2000*) Being Singular Plural*, Stanford: Stanford University Press.

Noether, Emmy (1918) "Invariant Variational Problems", in Yvette Kosmann Schwarzbach (ed.) and Bertram E. Schwarzbach (transl.), *The Noether Theorems. Invariance and Conservation Laws in the Twentieth Century*, New York: Springer.

Osiński, Zbigniew (1986) *Grotowski and His Laboratory*, New York: PAJ Publications.

Ostermeier, Thomas (1999) "Thomas Ostermeier im Interview", *Theater der Zeit* 4, 13.

Oswald, Genevieve (1983) "Myth and Legend in Martha Graham's 'Night Journey'", *Dance Research Annual* 14, 42–49.

Perloff, Marjorie (1991) *Radical Artifice. Writing Poetry in the Age of Media*, Chicago: University of Chicago Press.

Phelps, Lyon (1967) "Brecht's Antigone at the Living Theatre", *The Drama Review* 12:1, 125–131.

Piscator, Erwin (1980) *The Political Theatre*, London: Methuen.

Rae, Paul (2009) *Theatre and Human Rights*, London: Palgrave.

Rainer, Yvonne (1974) *Yvonne Rainer. Work 1961–73*, New York: Press of Nova Scotia College.

Rangacharya, Adya (1986) *Natyasastra*, Bangalore: IBH Prakashana.

Reynolds, Dee and Matthew Reason (2007) *Rhythmic Subjects. Uses of Energy in the Dances of Mary Wigman, Martha Graham and Merce Cunningham,* Hampshire: Dance Books.

——— (2012) *Kinesthetic Empathy in Creative and Cultural Practices*, Bristol: Intellect.

Richards, Thomas——— (1995) *At Work With Grotowski on Physical Actions*, London & New York: Routledge.

——— (2008) *Heart of Practice. Within the Workcenter of Jerzy Grotowski and Thomas Richard,* London & New York: Routledge.

Riencourt, Amaury de (1980) *The Eye of Shiva. Eastern Mysticism and Science*, London: Souvenir Press.

Roach, Joseph (1996) *Cities of the Dead. Circum-Atlantic Performance*, New York: Columbia University Press.

Romanyshyn, Robert D (2002) *Ways of the Heart. Essays towards an Imaginal Psychology*, Pittsburgh: Trivium Publications

Rose, David (2006) *Consciousness. Philosophical, Psychological and Neural Theories*, Oxford: Oxford University Press.

Ross, Janice (2007) *Anne Halprin. Experience as Dance*, Berkeley: University of California Press.

Roth, Moira (1977) "The Aesthetics of Indifference", *Artforum* 16:3, 46–53.

Said, Edward (1978) *Orientalism*, London: Routledge.

——— (1994) *Culture and Imperialism*, London: Vintage.

Salman, Sherry (2008) "The Creative Psyche: Jung's Major Contributions", in Polly Young-Eisendrath and Terence Dawson (eds.), *The Cambridge Companion to Jung*, Cambridge: Cambridge University Press, pp. 57–75.

Sanchez-Colberg, Ana (1996) "Altered States and Subliminal Spaces: Charting the Road towards a Physical Theatre", *Performance Research* 1:2, 40–56.

Sanders, Lorna (2007) "I Just Can't Wait to Get to the Hotel: Zero Degrees (2005)", http://www.akramkhancompany.net/html/akram_essay.php?id=16, accessed 23 July 2012.

Santos Newhall, Mary Anne (2009) *Mary Wigman*, London and New York: Routledge.

Sapir, Michael (2008) "Phase Shifting: Focus on Rosas", *Dance Theatre Journal* 22:3, 27–30.

Savarese, Nicola (2001) "1931. Antonin Artaud Sees Balinese Theatre at the Paris Colonial Exposition", *The Drama Review* 45:3, 51–77.

Sayama, Mike (1986) *Samadhi. Self-Development in Zen, Swordsmanship, and Psychotherapy*, New York: SUNY Press.

Schechner, Richard (1970) *Dionysus in 69: The Performance Group*, New York: Farrar, Strauss.

——— (1985) *Between Theater and Anthropology*, Philadelphia: University of Pennsylvania Press.

——— (1994) *Environmental Theatre*, London & New York: Applause Books.

——— (2001) "Rasaesthetics", *The Drama Review* 45:3, 27–50.

Scheer, Edward (2004) *Antonin Artaud. A Critical Reader*, London & New York: Routledge.

Schlagenwerth, Michaela (2008) *Sasha Waltz*, Berlin: Alexander Verlag.

Schlicher, Suzanne (1993) "The West German Dance Theatre", *Choreography and Dance* 3:2, 25–43.

Schmidt, Jochen (2002) *Tanzgeschichte des 20. Jahrhunderts in einem Band: 101 Choreografenporträts*, Berlin: Henschel.

Schneckenburger, Manfred (2007) *Antony Gormley. Bodies in Space*, Berlin: Bernhard Heiliger Stiftung.

Schwarz, Arturo (2000) *The Complete Works of Marcel Duchamp*, New York: Harry N. Abrams.

Seibert, Brian (2006) "The In-Between Place", *The Threepenny Review* 107, 17–18.

Sennet, Richard (2008) *The Craftsman*, London: Penguin.

Servos, Norbert (1998) "Pina Bausch: Dance and Emancipation", in Alexandrea Carter (ed.), *The Routledge Dance Studies Reader*, London and New York: Routledge, pp. 36–45.

——— (2008) *Pina Bausch Dance Theatre*, Munich: Kieser.

Sheets-Johnstone (2009) *The Corporeal Turn. An Interdisciplinary Reader*, Exeter: Imprint Academic.

Shephard, William Hunter (1991) *The Dionysus Group*, New York: Peter Lang.

Sloat, Susanna (2002) *Caribbean Dance from Abakuá to Zouk. How Movement Shapes Identity*, Gainesville, FL: University of Florida Press.

Sloman, Albert E (1950) *The Sources of Calderón's El Príncipe Constante*, Oxford: Blackwell.

Slowiak, James and Jairo Cuesta (2007) *Jerzy Grotowski*, London & New York: Routledge.

Soneji, Davesh, ed. (2010) *Bharatanatyam. A Reader*, Oxford: Oxford University Press.

Sophocles (1990) *Antigone. In a version by Bertolt Brecht*, transl. Judith Malina, New York: Applause Books.

Sörgel, Sabine (2007) *Dancing Postcolonialism: The National Dance Theatre Company of Jamaica*, Bielefeld: Transcript.

Soyinka, Wole (1993) *Death and the King's Horseman*, London: Methuen.

——— (1999) *The Burden of Memory, The Muse of Forgiveness*, Oxford: Oxford University Press.

Srinivasan, Priya (2012) *Sweating Saris: Indian Dance as Transnational Labor*, Philadelphia: Temple University Press.

States, Bert O. (1985) *Great Reckonings in Little Rooms. On the Phenomenology of Theatre*, Berkeley: University of California Press.

Stevens, Anthony (1994) *Jung. A Very Short Introduction*, Oxford: Oxford University Press.

Stevenson, Nick (2005) "Media, Cultural Citizenship and the Global Public Sphere", in Randall D. Germain and Michael Kenny (eds.), *The Idea of Global Civil Society. Politics and Ethics in a Globalizing Era*, London and New York: Routledge, pp. 67–83.

Stocker, Karl, Nadia Cusimano and Katia Schurl (2003) *Inside Out*, Wien: Springer Verlag.

Styan, J. L. (1981) *Modern Drama in Theory and Practice 3. Expressionism and Epic Theatre*, Cambridge: Cambridge University Press.

Sulcas, Roslyn (1992) "Space and Energy", *Dance and Dancers* April, pp. 13–17.

Szporer, Philip (2009) "Sidi Larbi Cherkaoui's *Sutra*: Awake in the World", http://www.hour.ca/2009/11/05/awake-in-the-world/, accessed 24 July 2012.

Tacey, David (2006) *How to Read Jung*, London: Granta Books.

Thompson Drewal, Margaret (2003) "Improvisation as Participatory Performance. Egungun Masked Dancers in the Yoruba Tradition", in Ann Cooper Albright and David Gere (eds.), *Taken by Surprise: A Dance Improvisation Reader*, Middletown, CT: Wesleyan University Press.

Thompson, Robert F. (1974) *African Art in Motion. Icon and Act*, Los Angeles: University of California Press.

Thoms, Victoria (2013) *Martha Graham: Gender and the Haunting of a Dance Pioneer*, Bristol: Intellect.

Toepfer, Karl (1997) *Empire of Ecstasy. Nudity and Movement in German Body Culture, 1910–1935*, Berkeley: University of California Press.

Tracy, Robert (1986) "Noguchi: Collaborating with Graham", *Ballet Review* 13, 9–17.

Turner, Victor (1969) *The Ritual Process. Structure and Anti-Structure*, New York: Aldine Publishing.

——— (1982) *From Ritual to Theatre. The Human Seriousness of Play*, ed. Brooks McNamara and Richard Schechner, New York: Performing Arts Journal Publications.

——— (1990) "Are There Universals of Performance in Myth, Ritual, and Drama?", in Richard Schechner and W. Appel (eds.), *By Means of Performance*, New York: Routledge, pp. 1–18.

Tytell, John (1997) *The Living Theatre. Art, Exile, and Outrage*, London: Methuen.

Uytterhoeven, Michel (2002) "Une couleur différente pour chaque nouvel horizon: la dimension international du travail de Rosas", in *Rosas/ Anne Teresa De Keersmaeker*, Tournai: La Renaissance du Livre.

Vivekananda, Swami (1914) *Raja Yoga*, Calcutta: Udbodhan Office.

Waldenfels, Bernard (2011) *Phenomenology of the Alien*, Evanston: Northwestern University Press.

Weigel, Helene, ed. (1952) *Theaterarbeit 6 Aufführungen des Berliner Ensembles*, Dresden: VVV Dresdener Verlag.

Weiss, Peter (2006) *Marat/Sade The Persecution and Assassination of Marat as Performed by the Inmates of the Asylum of Charenton under the direction of the Marquis de Sade*, London: Boyars.

Welsh-Asante, Kariamu (1996) *African Dance: An Artistic, Historical, and Philosophical Inquiry*, Trenton, NJ: Africa World Press.

——— (2001) "Commonalities in African Dance: An Aesthetic Foundation", in Ann Dills and Ann Cooper-Albright (eds.), *Moving History/ Dancing Cultures*, Middletown, CT: Wesleyan University Press, pp. 144–151.

Wiles, David (2000) *Greek Theatre Performance. An Introduction*, Cambridge: Cambridge University Press.

Wiles, Timothy J. (1980) *The Theatre Event. Modern Theories of Performance*, Chicago & London: University of Chicago Press.

Willett, John, ed. (1964) *Brecht on Theatre. The Development of an Aesthetic*, London: Methuen.

Winet, Evan (1998) "Great Reckonings in a Simulated City. Artaud's Misunderstanding of Balinese Theatre", *Crosscurrents in the Drama East and West* 6, Alabama: Alabama University Press, pp. 98–107.

Wolf, Naomi (2012) *Vagina. A New Biography*, London: Virago.

Wood, Catherine (2007) *The Mind is a Muscle*, London: Afterall Books.

Worth, Libby and Helen Poynor (2004) *Anne Halprin*, London and New York: Routledge.

Young-Eisendrath, Polly and Terence Dawson, eds. (2008) *The Cambridge Companion to Jung*, 2nd ed., Cambridge: Cambridge University Press.

——— (2008) "Jung and Buddhism: Refining the Dialogue", in Polly Young-Eisendrath and Terence Dawson (eds.), *The Cambridge Companion to Jung*, Cambridge: Cambridge University Press, pp. 235–251.

Zeltzer, Charles T. (2011) "The Wisdom of the Body in Kundalini, Alchemy and Individuation", *Guildpaper* No. 307, London: The Guild of Pastoral Psychology.

DVDs, Websites, and Other Media

Acocella, Joan (2009) "Martha Graham on Film", http://www.criterion.com/current/posts/615, accessed 15 September 2009.

Ailey, Alvin (2010) *An Evening with the Alvin Ailey American Dance Theatre*, 108 mins, Arthaus Musik.

Bausch, Pina (1984) *Blaubart. Beim Anhören einer Tonbandaufnahme von Béla Bartóks Oper "Herzog Blaubarts Burg"*, Live Recording at Opernhaus Wuppertal, Suhrkamp Verlag Production.

Brook, Peter (1967) *Marat/Sade*, 116 mins, colour, United Artists.

Cherkaoui, Sidi Larbi (2008a) *Sutra*, Live Recording at Sadler's Wells, 71 mins, colour, Axiom Films.

Cunningham, Merce (1973) *Walkaround Time*, 48 mins, colour, Electronic Arts Intermix.

DeMey, Thierry and Anne Teresa De Keersmaeker (2002) *Rosas Danst Rosas. A film by Thierry De Mey. Based on the choreography by Anne Teresa De Keersmaeker*, 1997, 57 mins, coulour.

Graham, Martha (1957) "A Dancer's World", Martha Graham Dance on Film: The Criterion Collection [2007], 31 mins, black and white.

——— (1961) "Night Journey", *Martha Graham Dance on Film: The Criterion Collection* [2007], 29 mins, black and white.

Halprin, Anne (2004) "Parades and Changes" and "Intensive Care", Excerpts from performances at Festival d'Automne Paris.

Jones, Bill T. and Arnie Zane Dance Company (2004) *Bill T Jones: Dancing to the Promised Land*, 60 mins, colour, BBC Documentary Production.

Kent, Don and Christian Dumais-Lvowski (2009) *Sidi Larbi Cherkaoui: Dreams of Babel*, 59 mins, colour, Bel Air.

Khan, Akram and Sidi Larbi Cherkaoui (2008) *Zero Degrees*, Live Recording at Sadler's Wells, 66 mins, colour, Axiom Films.

Malina, Judith and Julian Beck (1980) *The Living Theatre's Antigone*, 137 mins, black and white, Italian TV Production.

Schechner, Richard (1970) *Dionysus in 69*, 1h25min16′, black and white, Richard Schechner's Productions Collections, http://hidvl.nyu.edu/video/000031372_enhanced.html.

Shaolin Blogspot UK, http://shaolincity.blogspot.co.uk.

Themelis, Konstantinos (1986) *Conversations with Ryszard Cieslak*, Recording, Athens, Transcript Grotowski Archive University of Kent.

Waltz, Sasha and Guests (2011) *Körper/S/nobody*, Anniversary Edition, 210 mins, colour, Arthaus Musik.

Index